Praise for *Business Basics for Nurses*

"Today's healthcare environment needs nurses to lead innovation strategies that solve complex issues related to escalating healthcare costs, diminishing quality, and improving safety. Business Basics for Nurses *is a tool that can equip nurses with advanced knowledge in business skills, especially those who seek to further their careers to lead in the healthcare environment as well as those who seek to create their own innovative businesses. Written by Suzanne Waddill-Goad, a nurse who has been a successful businesswoman herself, this book guides nurses through the steps to becoming a successful business-minded nurse!"*

–Victoria Niederhauser, DrPH, RN, PPCNP-BC, FAAN
Dean & Professor, University of Tennessee Knoxville

"As a coaching and consulting business owner with 20 years' experience, I can attest to the value of this unique book. Business Basics for Nurses *addresses potential opportunities and common challenges, providing rich business resources for both the novice and experienced nurse entrepreneur. The writing is clear and conversational. Each chapter weaves together important concepts that leave the reader with inspiration, new knowledge, encouragement, and action steps to pursue a business venture. Chock-full of meaningful and practical business nuggets, it's a must-read for APNs, consultants, and leaders in a variety of settings."*

–Kimberly McNally, MN, RN, BCC
President, McNally & Associates

"This is a perfect book for nurses starting out as a healthcare manager or executive and for those who need to develop skills to start their own business. With her passion, positive energy, and knowledge, the author and her contributors make this book a fun read that provides the knowledge needed for success in the business world."

–Pamela D. Hardesty, PhD, RN, NEA-BC
Associate Clinical Professor, Concentration Coordinator,
MSN-Nursing Administration
College of Nursing, University of Tennessee, Knoxville

"Business Basics for Nurses *should be required reading in any nursing program. It will greatly assist in advancing students' budding understanding of the business of healthcare. This book fills a critical gap in nursing education."*

–Glen Lyon, MSN, RN
Urgent Care and Occ Med Manager, Sutter Health

BUSINESS BASICS
FOR NURSES

Suzanne Waddill-Goad,
DNP, MBA, RN, CEN

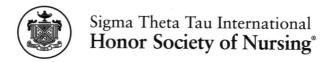

Sigma Theta Tau International
Honor Society of Nursing®

The Honor Society of Nursing, Sigma Theta Tau International (STTI) is a nonprofit organization whose mission is advancing world health and celebrating nursing excellence in scholarship, leadership, and service. Founded in 1922, STTI has more than 135,000 active members in over 90 countries and territories. Members include practicing nurses, instructors, researchers, policymakers, entrepreneurs, and others. STTI's 520 chapters are located at more than 700 institutions of higher education throughout Armenia, Australia, Botswana, Brazil, Canada, Colombia, England, Ghana, Hong Kong, Japan, Jordan, Kenya, Lebanon, Malawi, Mexico, the Netherlands, Pakistan, Philippines, Portugal, Singapore, South Africa, South Korea, Swaziland, Sweden, Taiwan, Tanzania, Thailand, the United States, and Wales. Learn more at www.nursingsociety.org.

Sigma Theta Tau International
550 West North Street
Indianapolis, IN, USA 46202

To order additional books, buy in bulk, or order for corporate use, contact Nursing Knowledge International at 888.NKI.4YOU (888.654.4968/US and Canada) or +1.317.634.8171 (outside US and Canada).

To request a review copy for course adoption, email solutions@nursingknowledge.org or call 888. NKI.4YOU (888.654.4968/US and Canada) or +1.317.634.8171 (outside US and Canada).

To request author information, or for speaker or other media requests, contact Marketing, Honor Society of Nursing, Sigma Theta Tau International at 888.634.7575 (US and Canada) or +1.317.634.8171 (outside US and Canada).

ISBN: 9781940446189
EPUB ISBN: 9781940446196
PDF ISBN: 9781940446202
MOBI ISBN: 9781940446219

Library of Congress Cataloging-in-Publication data

Names: Waddill-Goad, Suzanne, author. | Sigma Theta Tau International, issuing body.
Title: Business basics for nurses / Suzanne Waddill-Goad.
Description: Indianapolis, IN : Sigma Theta Tau International, [2017] | Description based on print version record and CIP data provided by publisher; resource not viewed.
Identifiers: LCCN 2017021067 (print) | LCCN 2017021690 (ebook) | ISBN 9781940446196 (Epub) | ISBN 9781940446202 (Pdf) | ISBN 9781940446219 (Mobi) | ISBN 9781940446189 (print : alk. paper) | ISBN 9781940446219 (mobi)
Subjects: | MESH: Economics, Nursing | Practice Management | United States
Classification: LCC RT86.7 (ebook) | LCC RT86.7 (print) | NLM WY 77 | DDC 610.73068--dc23
LC record available at https://lccn.loc.gov/2017021067

First Printing, 2017

Publisher: Dustin Sullivan
Acquisitions Editor: Emily Hatch
Editorial Coordinator: Paula Jeffers
Cover Designer: Rebecca Batchelor
Interior Design/Page Layout: Rebecca Batchelor

Principal Book Editor: Carla Hall
Development and Project Editor: Kate Shoup
Copy Editor: Charlotte Kughen
Proofreader: Erin Geile
Indexer: Larry D. Sweazy

Dedication

This book is dedicated to those who first sparked my interest in learning about the business of healthcare: Mr. Michael Tuohy, Mr. Thomas Nielsen, Mr. Mike Bonthuis, Mrs. Linda Garner, Ms. Jane Bailey, Mrs. Marie Smith (and the consulting team at APM), Dr. Ruth Hansten, and Mr. Michael Porter.

Acknowledgments

This book would not have been possible without the dedicated publishing team at STTI, as well as three nurse colleagues who wrote about their experiences in the business of healthcare as contributors: Dr. Anna Kiger, Dr. Holly Langster, and Dr. Charlotte Mason. The contributors' vast experience and diverse expertise made this book better.

Thank you, too, to my family and friends who provided encouragement when the going got tough and time was in short supply.

Finally, thank you to my readers. I hope they enjoy this book about business. Over the last decade, I have discovered that I really like writing. It provides an outlet to share professional and life experiences, as well as a venue to be heard.

About the Author

Suzanne Waddill-Goad, DNP, MBA, RN, CEN

Before founding her own consulting practice in 2003, Dr. Waddill-Goad held the positions of chief nursing officer/assistant administrator, operations improvement coordinator, director of quality improvement, hospital supervisor, and charge nurse. As a staff nurse, she chose to work both as an employee and a temporary nurse in hospital and physician office settings with work assignments of varying duration in a multitude of clinical areas.

Suzanne's graduate education was focused in executive and managerial leadership. She holds a doctor of nursing practice (DNP) in executive leadership from American Sentinel University, a master of business administration (with a specialty in managerial leadership) from City University of Seattle, and a bachelor of science in nursing from the University of Colorado. She continues to maintain her clinical certification in emergency nursing and completed an Executive Education Certificate in Lean Six Sigma (Black Belt) from The Ohio State University, Fisher College of Business in 2009.

In 2014, Suzanne received a faculty appointment to the University of Tennessee in Knoxville, Tennessee as an assistant clinical professor. She has since taught for both the College of Nursing and the Haslam College of Business in their executive education programs. In 2016, she published her first book, *Nurse Burnout: Overcoming Stress in Nursing*.

Suzanne is a results-oriented nurse leader committed to finding the most optimal solutions to the challenges that healthcare providers, clinicians, and facilities face in their efforts to balance cost and quality, while providing excellent service and superior clinical outcomes.

About the Contributors

Charlotte Kearney Mason, DNP, MS, APRN, is a board-certified family nurse practitioner and the owner of Jackson Whole Family Health in Jackson, Wyoming. A pioneer for independent, nurse practitioner, patient-centered care, she opened her practice in 2002. In addition to her clinical practice, Dr. Mason is a founding member of the Teton Free Clinic and continues to serve as a board member.

As a clinical preceptor, Charlotte mentors nurses and advance practice nursing students from universities across the country. She has presented on the topic of diabetes care in the elderly for the Sigma Theta Tau International Nursing Research Congress, the Utah Diabetes Association, and the Frontiers in Wyoming Medicine conference.

Charlotte holds a doctor of nursing practice (DNP) degree from the University of Utah, a master of science (MS) and an advance practice registered nurse (APRN) degree from the University of Wyoming, and a bachelor of science in nursing (BSN) degree from the University of Colorado. Charlotte is the mother of three beautiful and independent girls, a skier, and a long-distance triathlete.

Holly Langster, DNP, FNP-C, HCA, CENP, is a nurse practitioner from Heber Springs, Arkansas. Dr. Langster works at the Myeloma Institute at the University of Arkansas for Medical Sciences in Little Rock, Arkansas as the executive director for clinical operations. Holly owns and operates her own business, Beauty Refinement by Holly, offering cosmetic procedures such as Botox and cosmetic fillers, as well as laser hair removal and skin treatments. Holly also works with attorneys across the state of Arkansas to assist with nursing review of medical legal cases.

As a partner with a medical director, Holly helped build the Breast Center at SIU in Springfield, Illinois. As a nurse practitioner, Holly learned the specialty practice of caring for and managing patients with a variety of breast diseases, including cancer. Administratively, Holly worked to ensure that the operations of the Breast Center were efficient and effective, and with the team approach to the fight against breast disease, the center eventually grew into the Cancer Institute of SIU. Nursing administration became a larger focus as Holly moved south to Arkansas and began working with the Baptist Health System, where more than a decade in healthcare administration expanded her exposure to hospital management and operations.

Holly holds a doctor of nursing practice in executive leadership from American Sentinel University, a master in healthcare administration from Southern Illinois University, a master's degree in nursing as a family nurse practitioner from the University of Illinois at Chicago, a bachelor of science in nursing from Bradley University, and a nursing diploma from Methodist Medical School of Nursing. She is board certified as a family nurse practitioner and as an executive nursing leader.

Her husband is an emergency room physician, and they have one child, Lucas. Holly is the daughter of an RN, the granddaughter of an LPN, and the great-granddaughter of the town midwife. She believes that nurses need a good foundation in business if they aspire to work administratively or independently.

Anna J. Kiger, DNP, DSc, MBA, NEA-BC, RN, is the chief nurse officer and system vice president for Sutter Health, a not-for-profit healthcare system operating in Northern California and the San Francisco Bay Area. Prior to her current position, Anna was the system chief nurse officer and vice president of patient care services for Tenet Health Care, an $18 billion for-profit health system based in Dallas, Texas. As the system chief nursing officer (CNO), Anna was responsible for the nursing operations of 81 acute-care hospitals stretched across 16 states.

During her 16-year tenure at Tenet, Anna worked with colleagues to design a system-wide approach to healthcare operations in areas such as quality, safety, growth, and cost. She is very proud of the eight hospitals that achieved Magnet or Pathway to Excellence designations, which recognize excellence in nursing practice and patient outcomes. Before joining Tenet in 1999, Anna was the associate vice president for nursing at Tulane University Hospital & Clinics in New Orleans, Louisiana, a

342-bed academic medical center owned by HCA Corporation, a for-profit healthcare system. At Tulane, she was responsible for a nursing staff of more than 650 full-time employees.

Anna received her undergraduate nursing degree from West Virginia University School of Nursing in Morgantown, West Virginia; a master of science in nursing administration from Duquesne University; a master in business from Averett University; a doctor of science in public health, health systems management from Tulane School of Public Health & Tropical Medicine; and a doctor of nursing practice from Texas Tech University School of Nursing.

Anna is a member of the editorial boards for the *Journal of Nursing Administration* (*JONA*) and the American Society for Healthcare Risk Management's *Journal of Healthcare Risk Management*.

Her husband Earl is a former hospital controller. She has two children, Grace and Wesley. Her first grandchild is on the way.

Table of Contents

Foreword

Business and nursing. These two words seem to contradict each other. Nursing is synonymous with adjectives like caring, compassion, warmth, kindness, competence, and safety—and for years has been the most trusted profession (Gallup, 2016). Business is notoriously stereotyped as cruel, cutthroat, fast-paced, and self-centered. Yet healthcare systems are businesses, and many nurses are thrown into management positions early in their careers without any business knowledge.

When I graduated from nursing school in the early 1990s, my plan was to work as a clinician for a few years and then go back to school and become a nurse practitioner. During that time, the payment system in healthcare was changing from a fee-for-service model to a managed care model. Diagnosis-related groups (DRGs) became the standard payment method. This change caused chaos. Revenue declined significantly, and health systems across the country were forced to reduce costs to remain solvent. Because labor is typically the highest expense in healthcare, organizations began flattening management structures and increasing the span and scope of many leaders. My organization was no different.

I remember the turning point of my nursing career, when my director asked me to apply for an assistant director position during the payment-system changes. I hesitated, knowing this was not my career path, but I eventually gave in with one condition: I could go back to bedside nursing if I didn't like it.

Once in the new job, I quickly realized that I lacked critical business knowledge. I knew how to balance my checkbook and manage my home, but I did not have the skills or knowledge to manage my department, the budget, the financial statements, and the daily operations. I decided the best way to learn was to step outside of healthcare and immerse myself in the business world. With a little help from my first husband, who said, "You'll never make it in the business world," I enrolled in a non-healthcare master of business administration (MBA) program. This was a huge win that propelled me into executive leadership and opened my world to many of the concepts and ideas you will read about in this book.

Fast forward to 2010. I had the opportunity to enroll in a doctor of nursing practice (DNP) program. Because I had an MBA rather than a master of science in nursing (MSN), I had to take a few prerequisite courses before starting the actual program—including a course titled "Nursing Theory." This is when I met my dear friend Suzanne (Suzi) Waddill-Goad, the author of this book. We had very similar career paths as we both chose the MBA instead of the MSN route, were executive nursing leaders, and had a continued desire to translate our knowledge into practice. Neither one of us was thrilled to go back to Nursing 101, but in retrospect it provided some levity to our intense work as executives while grounding us, again, in the foundational aspects of our role as nurse leaders.

As you read this book, you'll see that Suzi has used both her nursing and business background in most aspects of her career. During our DNP program, she was known as the "idea girl." Some of those ideas were far-reaching, some of them walked the edge, and others were just plain fun! (Some secrets I won't tell.) No matter how impossible the task ahead seemed, Suzi brought humor, optimism, and enthusiasm to the table.

Healthcare is now going through yet another transformation. The complexity of services, definition of value, and intensity of payment reform are just a few topics on the agenda. Blending the science of nursing and business is no longer an oxymoron—it is a necessity. *Business Basics for Nurses* provides a valuable resource for nurses not only in leadership, but also those at the bedside who are ultimately driving the value proposition for healthcare.

–Kristin Schmidt, DNP, MBA, RN, NEA-BC, CENP, CPHQ, FACHE
Chief Nursing Officer, Tenet Healthcare
Fountain Valley Regional Hospital and Medical Center
Fountain Valley, California

Introduction

Welcome to *Business Basics for Nurses*. This book aims to deliver a "prescription" for nurses—one that will cure them of their unfamiliarity with the basics of business.

Why write a book about business for nurses? Because business *is* the foundation of healthcare. What goes on behind the scenes, beyond caring for patients, is just as important as clinical care. If you think of all the people who work in nearly any healthcare entity, only a portion of them provide clinical care. It is all of the non-clinical people who set the stage: Negotiating contracts with payers (to obtain patients), registration and collections (creating a paper trail and starting the revenue cycle), purchasing supplies (for clinicians and others to use), ordering equipment (to accomplish work), locating real estate (to conduct the business), setting organizational policy and procedure, leading the team (senior level leadership), accounting (managing the flow of money), and so on.

The phone directory in any healthcare entity is a good way to actually see how many people and departments it takes to provide healthcare! What do nurses need to know about business? It would be wise to learn everything you can. It will make you a much more valuable employee if you have an understanding of the merit that those who support your work provide. A successful business is always made up of a thousand little things: leadership, committed employees, balancing risk, sound decision-making, action, a passion for the mission and vision, values, purpose, and a little luck.

Rishel (2014) argues that business acumen is crucial for nurses. She believes that whether nurses work on the front lines, in leadership positions, or in research, it is imperative they understand the business of healthcare. This extends far beyond the need to control cost; understanding the supply chain, the global cost of care, quality initiatives, and intricate financial aspects all add to a nurse's knowledge and enable her to determine how best to care for others using evidence for best practices and relevant research in a responsible way. With this book, you will discover how knowledge of all these "little things" can help you in your nursing career.

> *"If opportunity doesn't knock,*
> *build a door."*
> –Milton Berle

What Exactly Is Business?

Business is defined as "an organization or economic system where goods and services are exchanged for another or money" (Business, n.d.). Business makes things happen around the world and affects nearly all parts of our society. It really does make the world turn. Without it, what would we all be doing? Most people don't think about what business is and how it actually works. A more simplified definition is that it encompasses the wide-ranging development and delivery of all global products and services—including healthcare.

Take produce for example. Someone has to procure and prep the land to plant seeds or plants, care for the growth material, and then harvest the product. There must be customer demand for the final product—produce—and it must be transported to reach those customers. In other words, people must both want it and be able to buy it. Each of these steps provides an opportunity for business: selling land, prepping land, generating seeds or plants, setting up the area for growth, providing fertilizer and pesticide control (if not an organic operation) for the growth material, caretaking of the plants, harvesting, selling or distributing the final product, and obtaining customers and sales.

A contrasting healthcare example could be a patient who presents with an emergency to a hospital. He arrives and must be registered (at some time, depending on the level of severity of his injury or illness), and clinicians must quickly assess his medical need and determine treatment options. All pertinent data are entered into the patient's health record. Once treated, the patient is educated about his condition, counseled on follow up treatment, and released. Many of the things nurses may not consider is someone had to purchase the land, design the building, obtain permits, construct the space, order equipment and supplies, test the equipment and building systems, set up the infrastructure of the systems for information flow (vendor contracts, registration, billing, ordering, collections, implementing the electronic health record, etc.), clean the building and ready it for operation (as well as maintenance), hire the personnel of all types to run the entity, buy food and prepare it, manage

You've probably sat through the safety announcements on a flight. As part of those announcements, flight attendants advise passengers that in the event of an emergency, if the oxygen masks descend, everyone should put on their own oxygen mask before assisting others. The same could be said in business, especially if you are in a leadership role. You must take care of yourself to be at your best to care for others. As simple as this sounds, most people don't do it!

the flow of money and investments, etc. Hospitals and most any health entity are a complex web of systems.

As a child, I developed an early curiosity about business and how things worked while scheming to open my first lemonade stand. First, I had to convince my parents that it was a viable idea. But that wasn't all. There were so many questions to consider—questions that, I would come to learn, could apply to almost any business venture:

- **What day of the week might be best for sales?** This, I later discovered, was a matter of sales, marketing, and business intelligence.

- **What time of day would be best for sales?** This, too, was a matter of sales, marketing, and business intelligence.

- **What should I charge?** Answering this question came from information gleaned through market and competitive research.

- **Were there any other similar businesses (in my case, lemonade stands) in the area?** This was also a matter of market and competitive research.

- **Where should the business be located for the best exposure?**

> The difference between entrepreneurism and intraprenuerism is simply the level of risk one is willing to take. Venturing outside your comfort zone and the relative safety of being employed within an organization takes guts!

Again, market and competitive research applied. So, too, did location research.

- **How sweet should the product (lemonade) be?** Of course, this wouldn't apply to every product. But for those it *does* apply to, it would fall under the category of recipes and trade secrets.

- **How fancy should the location (lemonade stand) be?** This was a simple matter of the cost of materials and startup costs.

- **How much will it cost me to make the product (lemonade) and set up the location (lemonade stand)?** This, too, was related to the cost of materials and startup costs, as well as cash flow.

- **Will customers keep coming back?** This was all about customer satisfaction.

- **Will they tell their friends, neighbors, and family members that my product (lemonade) was good and urge them to come try it?** The answer to this question related to marketing via customer satisfaction.

- **What would happen if so many people came that I ran out?**
  Here, the issue was product satisfaction and supply chain.

The answers to these questions were valuable. Each one represented prized information, enabling me to make my business even better.

I didn't stop at my lemonade stand, however. What followed were many other experimental business ventures for whatever I was into at the time. I was and continue to be an "idea girl." Each opportunity proved to be excellent training in business-related skills, especially with regard to developing creative ideas and innovative approaches to problem-solving, forming and analyzing plans, setting goals, and perfecting my skills in sales and negotiation. Each of these would be so useful to me later in life! When I worked as a clinical nurse, doctors said I could "sell ice to an Eskimo." As a nurse leader, I set and exceeded many goals. Since then, I have become the proud owner of several successful business ventures.

People have always told me that I am different, which I take as a compliment. They say that I think differently from the majority of people, that I am able to say things others cannot (such as delivering bad news) in an acceptable fashion, that I can implement creative solutions to complex problems, and that I always seem optimistic despite any negative organizational circumstances. As to the last point, cultivating and maintaining a healthy mind is paramount. There will be challenges and setbacks. Things won't always go as planned. Remaining flexible and even-tempered in the face of unpredictable circumstance separates successful leaders from those who are not—in business and in life. Grit and a positive mindset are vital attributes for success in business.

"It's not that we need new ideas,
but we need to stop having old ideas."
–Edwin Land

Do You Fit Inside or Outside an Organization?

Do you fit inside or outside an organization? Put another way, are you an *intra*preneur or an *entre*preneur? An *entrepreneur* is someone who is willing to start a business and risk loss in order to make money (Entrepreneur, n.d.). *Intrapreneurs* are typically managers within an organization who are able to influence and promote new services, products, and marketing (Intrapreneur, n.d.).

Although intrapreneurs work within an organization and entrepreneurs do not, their way of thinking is virtually the same. Both intrapreneurs and entrepreneurs are needed now more than ever. Business is fraught with uncertainty, changing conditions, and challenging situations that both intrapreneurs and entrepreneurs must be able to navigate confidently. This is especially true in healthcare, as there is no shortage of problems to solve.

SEVEN TIPS FOR ENTREPRENEURS

Wang (2016) cites seven tips from one of the most successful female entrepreneurs of all time, Diane Hendricks from ABC Supply:

- **You can take many paths to get to the same place.** Flexibility is key to navigating daily challenges.

- **Think long and hard before you start.** You must plan and be passionate about the work.

- **Do your homework.** Research and obtain expert advice when necessary.

- **Not everyone will believe in your vision.** Persevere anyway.

- **Juggle family and business the best way you know how.** It takes commitment and sacrifice.

- **Grasp the chances that come your way.** Be opportunistic in your thinking.

- **Most importantly, don't quit.** You will make mistakes. When you do, keep going.

> *"Fail often so you can*
> *succeed sooner."*
> –Tom Kelley

What Defines Success?

What is the definition of success in business? It depends on who is asking. Success in business can be defined by myriad perspectives. However, one thing most successful people *do* agree on is that hard work and perseverance are crucial, despite setbacks or failure (DeMers, 2014a). Every business environment in every industry can be extremely tough.

> *"There's only one growth strategy:*
> *work hard."*
> –William Hague

Regardless of the type of business you may choose, achieving success requires a distinctive set of skills. You can obtain these skills through formal academic programming, from less-formal sources such as a variety of training programs, and via on-the-job learning in one or more professional roles.

> *"If you really look closely, most*
> *overnight successes took a long time."*
> –Steve Jobs

Dealing With Challenges

During the first year in my consulting career, a male chief executive officer (CEO) yelled at me during a meeting. Because I had not experienced this type of behavior in any leadership role or previous business setting, I was a bit taken aback. Shortly after the meeting, I called a mentor of mine to get her perspective on what had transpired. I was surprised to learn that she, too, had experienced the same type of behavior in her consulting practice. She explained that although it wasn't a daily occurrence, it did happen. She warned me that this was probably just the first of many more challenging situations of all types. Unfortunately, she was right. The next 2 decades of my career were fraught with difficult negotiations, gender bias, and many more situations in which leaders displayed bad behavior. I quickly learned that not everyone has the same frame of reference, business ethics, or tolerance for adversity. I also learned to set limits with my clients. I now expect professionalism and no longer tolerate bad behavior.

Regarding gender bias, whereas the nursing profession is essentially dominated by women, the business environment has historically been dominated by men. Not surprisingly, in my experience as both a hospital executive and as a consultant, I typically find myself negotiating with men. Sometimes, gender differences get in the way. These gender differences are often accentuated in business by differences of opinion, communication styles, and strategies to obtain results. Fortunately, however, the business environment is changing. As more women attend business school and move into significant leadership roles, including CEOs of both for-profit and non-profit companies, they have begun to infiltrate the business landscape.

WOMEN IN BUSINESS

Although there are still more men than women in business, women possess unique skills to be successful. Women are naturally insightful, intuitive, caring, and organized, all while being compassionate. Llopis (2011) described women as opportunity experts. They see the potential in everyone and everywhere. He also described women as adept at skills such as networking, caregiving, and relationships. If you think that sounds a little like the skills needed to be a good nurse, you're right. It follows, then, that nursing and business are a natural fit.

---

*"The only place success comes before
work is in the dictionary."*
–Vidal Sassoon

Assessing Readiness

Do you daydream about how things would be if *you* were in charge?
Are you always looking for ways to improve things? Do you think
creatively? Are you full of good ideas? Do you possess fortitude? Are
you resilient in the face of adversity? If you answered yes to any of these
questions, you may be ready for the challenges business can bring.

Certain personal traits also serve as predictors of readiness. In a blog
post on the website for the Minority Business Development Agency, a
division of the United States Department of Commerce, business startup
expert Jason Bowser (n.d.) cited the eight traits of successful entrepreneurs:

1. **They have leadership skills.**

    - They possess strong leader-like qualities.

    - They're open to learning. (The old adage, "Leaders are
      made, not born," is true!)

    - They value attaining the goal, despite any challenges
      along the way.

    - They're good communicators and can bring diverse
      groups together.

    - They are respected and trusted.

2. **They are self-motivated.**

    - They go out into the world and make change work for
      them.

    - They're creators, disrupters, and adapters.

- They have a clear vision and strong passion for their work.

3. **They have a strong sense of ethics and integrity.**

   - They know that cheaters and thieves may win in the short term, but they will always lose in the long term. Reputation is everything in business, and it's only as good as your last client or engagement.

   - They maintain the highest standards of integrity.

4. **They are willing to fail.**

   - They are not afraid to fail.

   - They are expert risk calculators.

   - Their motto is, "Nothing ventured, nothing gained."

5. **They are innovative.**

   - They welcome change.

   - They are driven by new ideas and making improvements.

6. **They are aware of what they don't know.**

   - They are rarely afraid to ask questions.

   - They believe they can always leverage insight and information for better decision-making.

   - They have a healthy amount of confidence.

7. **They have a competitive spirit.**

   - They enjoy a challenge and like to win.

8. **They understand the value of a strong peer network.**

   - They know that becoming a success in business is rarely a solo journey. It takes a network of contacts, business and financial partners, and peers.

   - They value having a strong team to surround them.

"Speed, quality, price: pick two."
—Anonymous, quoted in The Economist

Conclusion

This book is targeted toward nurses who seek to develop business skills. It outlines several situations and examples to cover the following topics:

- Setting up or assessing infrastructure

- Evaluating business processes

- Influences on the external and internal environments in healthcare

- Determining value

- Building business-related plans of various types

- Compliance

- Finance

- Leveraging technology

- Capitalizing on expertise

- Marketing

- Leadership

- Relevant nursing practice essentials and innovation

Each chapter contains special boxes with pithy thoughts, case studies, and/or real-world stories, as well as exercises for you to demonstrate mastery of the presented concepts. Chapters also include a unique "Concept Capture" feature, which highlights relevant concepts in the chapter's content using a variety of strategies, such as reflective questions, case studies or examples, mental exercises, and/or experiential learning with suggested experiments. Our hope is that these will help you to better learn and understand the book's key concepts.

Each of the contributors to this text have their own experiences in and with business: one as a self-employed nurse practitioner practicing family medicine in a rural but very busy vacation area, one as a nurse leader and self-employed cosmetic nurse practitioner practicing in the beauty-enhancement arena, and one as a system chief nurse executive who has worked both in for-profit and non-profit organizations setting policy and supervising practice for large numbers of nurses and other clinicians. If you're interested in learning about business, read on.

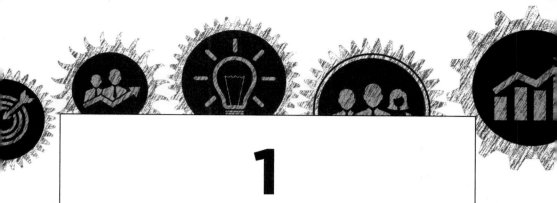

1

BUSINESS BASICS: THE BIG PICTURE IN HEALTHCARE

The World Bank Group (2016) describes *health expenditures* in general as the sum of all public and private monies spent related to healthcare. These include preventative and curative services; family-planning activities; nutritional counseling; and emergency aid. According to Fuchs (2013), following an analysis of the past 60 years, the growth rate of national healthcare expenditures appears to be closely related to the growth of the gross domestic product (GDP), thus tying the overall state of the economy to healthcare expansion or contraction. The GDP is a monetary measure of the total value of a nation's economy in a given time period, such as quarterly or annually (United States Department of Commerce, Bureau of Economic Analysis, 2016). In 2014, the U.S. GDP was estimated to be $17.42 trillion (The World Bank Group, 2016).

The External Environment

Healthcare in the U.S. is *big* business. Not only that, the industry is fraught with chaos due to governmental initiatives, political influence, and policy changes yet to be fully executed. This may explain why spending on healthcare in the United States far exceeds that of most other developed countries. In fact, healthcare spending represented 17.1% of the GDP (over one-sixth of it!) in 2014—approximately $2.96 trillion (The World Bank Group, 2014). Even so, disparities in healthcare access, benefit coverage, and specialty care remain.

A listing of the world's spending percentages of GDP for healthcare can be found at this link: http://data.worldbank.org/indicator/NY.GDP.PCAP.CD.

The high cost of healthcare isn't the only problem. Changing demographics present another challenge. In 2016, the World Bank Group cited 2015 U.S. population estimates at 321.21 million. Table 1.1 displays the age distribution for the U.S. population (as of 2014), as estimated by the Kaiser Family Foundation (2016). As shown in the table, the majority of the U.S. population is aging. With that comes an increase in both healthcare consumption and expenditures.

If you're interested in a more in-depth analysis of a specific geographic region, you can find state-by-state data at this link on the Kaiser Family Foundation's website: http://kff.org/other/state-indicator/distribution-by-age/.

TABLE 1.1 2014 U.S. AGE DISTRIBUTION							
Children 0-18	**Adults 19-25**	**Adults 26-34**	**Adults 35-44**	**Adults 45-54**	**Adults 55-64**	**Adults 65+**	**Total**
United States 25%	10%	12%	13%	13%	13%	15%	100%

©*Kaiser Family Foundation. Used with permission*

Both these factors—the high cost of healthcare in the U.S. coupled with the nation's aging population—indicate that the American healthcare industry is ripe for change. But who will lead that change? I posit that nurses are uniquely positioned to lead this change.

> *"In the midst of chaos,*
> *there is also opportunity."*
> –Sun Tzu, The Art of War

Nursing is healthcare's largest single profession. There are more than 3.1 million nurses in the U.S., with nearly 85% actively employed in the field (American Association of Colleges of Nursing [AACN], 2016). Nurses represent a mere 1% of the U.S. population, but are estimated to outnumber other medical providers by as many as four times, as described in a "Nursing Fact Sheet" by the American Association of Colleges of Nursing (AACN, 2011). For now, the majority (62.2% in 2008) are employed by hospitals (2011). As healthcare continues to evolve and the population ages, nursing jobs will continue to change, with new opportunities emerging in a variety of settings where care is or will be provided.

Nurses are smart people. We must step up and be willing to lead change. The current system of healthcare (or "sick care," as it might be more aptly called) needs it. The collective influence the profession could wield over systemic change is an untapped opportunity. Nurses could lead the charge to revolutionize and promote health, wellness, and the prevention of illness, both in and out of established organizations. To do so, however, nurses must continue to expand their responsibilities and to gain an understanding of aspects of healthcare that have historically been beyond their purview, including business. Perhaps this quote sums it up best (Rishel, 2014, p. 324):

> Understanding the relationship between the business of healthcare and the quality of care delivered to patients with cancer is not just for nurses in leadership positions. Implementing findings from research studies that describe best practices in cancer nursing is not just for nurse researchers. Improving outcomes and the quality of life for patients with cancer is a responsibility we all share.

The Internal Environment

In 2016, the number of registered hospitals in the U.S. was 5,627, according to the American Hospital Association Health Forum, LLC (2016). The number of hospitals has steadily declined in recent years as healthcare has changed. The American Hospital Association (AHA) profiles the number and types of hospitals on an annual basis; specific yearly data can be found here: http://www.aha.org/research/rc/stat-studies/fast-facts.shtml.

Economic pressures and the increasing complexity of reimbursement for hospital services have potentiated these closures. Indeed, according to the AHA (2016a), repeated cuts totaling nearly $136 billion in reimbursement have occurred at hospitals since 2010; and in 2014, hospitals received only $.89 in reimbursement for every dollar spent to provide services for Medicare patients and $.90 of reimbursement for every dollar spent caring for Medicaid patients. Medicare and Medicaid patients are estimated to total between 60 and 65% of a typical hospital's patient/payer mix (AHA, 2016b). The result in 2014 was a $51 billion underpayment gap (AHA, 2016b).

Cost pressures are seen in virtually every healthcare setting. Not surprisingly, they are also felt by nursing.

Even as reimbursement has declined, the cost to provide services has continually risen. This is a recipe for economic disaster. The complexity of pay for performance and clinical outcome–based reimbursement has also burdened the healthcare industry. Much of the pressure has come from payers as well as purchasers of healthcare services due to high cost.

> *"No margin, no mission."*
> *–Sister Irene Kraus, RN*

How much will be spent on healthcare in the next decade or two is anyone's guess. We do know, however, that future spending will likely be tied to the economy (as noted earlier in this chapter, in the discussion about GDP). It will also factor in the prevalence of chronic disease, such as obesity, infectious diseases, and dementia, as well as changes in medical technology, new drugs, new medical devices, imaging enhancements, and new surgical procedures, as described by Fuchs (2013) in the *New England Journal of Medicine*.

Given the high cost of healthcare and other economic pressures both now and in the future, it's clear that healthcare organizations can benefit from nurses who possess some business savvy—despite the fact that, as noted by Carlson (2015), nursing and business have historically been unlikely bedfellows (except for those in nursing leadership positions, who have been required to learn about various aspects of business). Changes in the industry require that nurses embrace finance and business acumen for improved practice. The areas for improvement are nearly endless. This list cites only a few:

- **Staffing:** Facilitate the appropriate use of available resources.

- **Supply selection:** Choose the correct supply for the task at hand.

- **Organization:** Become more organized to improve your and your unit's workflow.

- **Efficiency:** Become more efficient in your work by streamlining and/or eliminating steps in a process or tasks.

- **Downtime:** Use downtime productively to improve something in your work area.

- **Education:** Learn about finance via your practice or unit area's budget and performance.

"Creativity is thinking up new things. Innovation is doing new things."
–Theodore Levitt

THE HIGH COST OF LABOR

Generally, the largest cost in any healthcare operation is labor. In many organizations, nurses have felt the pain of staff reductions that have been made in an attempt to keep the organization(s) fiscally solvent. This also explains the rise of initiatives within organizations such as Lean, Six Sigma, high reliability, and other quality-improvement methodologies, as well as the shift of certain types of care from hospitals to outpatient settings.

This shift is expected to continue in the future, as is a renewed focus on the prevention of illness via a multitude of wellness programs. These initiatives will undoubtedly provide numerous employment choices for nurses in the future. There are hundreds (if not more) of non-hospital options for nursing employment, and that number is likely to grow. Consulting opportunities have likewise increased, with new specialties emerging nearly every day. And novel and creative specialties of medical practice—such as concierge medicine, where providers focus on the necessary steps for patients to stay well rather than simply treating illness—are evolving. Although it might seem counterintuitive for patients to visit their provider when well, this practice could decrease the overall consumption of healthcare resources and cost, while also improving patient-provider relationships and patient outcomes.

This shift in focus represents a radical change in thinking compared to the current system of healthcare in the U.S., and is a perfect fit for nursing in the future. Other positive changes in the healthcare industry will provide even more opportunities for nurses to practice in new and different ways.

A literature search revealed similar conversations in the United Kingdom and Australia about the importance of nurses gaining an understanding of business basics to drive necessary change.

Building a Value Proposition

A key tenet of business is the idea of *value*. Consulting guru Alan Weiss describes value as the importance, worth, and/or usefulness of a product or service (Weiss, 2016, p. 84). Hence, value is always determined by the customer. Payers and patients expect value for purchased services in the form of compassionate care. Excellence in service delivery and the quality of care are assumed to be the norm.

Savvy entrepreneurs and organizations know all about value. They strive to create value by solving problems and filling the gap between *want* and *need*. This is called a *value proposition*. Emerging organizations that effectively fill this gap include Uber, the ride-sharing service; AirBnB, which matches travelers with lodging provided by local hosts; and Trivago, the travel search service that uses many search engines at one time to find the best availability and pricing.

Opportunities to create value in healthcare are similarly plentiful. They might include providing certain types of services for elder or senior care, managing chronic illness, and other related services. Indeed, thanks to new technology, some improvements have already come to pass, such as billboards with emergency department wait times, applications (apps) for appointment scheduling, electronic access for patients to retrieve electronic medical records, and more.

According to an article by Seth Kahan (2013) in *Fast Company*, there are three ways to create value that lasts:

- **The creation of new value:** This might include breaking into a new sector, creating a new line of business, or creating market need for access to a new target market.

- **The creation or perception of more value:** This could involve adjusting pricing, giving more for the same pricing, or both.

- **The creation or delivery of better value:** This means expanding existing value by increasing quality, not quantity. This could be perceived by changes in impact, intensity, and/or application of a product or service.

Apple is an excellent example of a company that creates value. By designing computers, the iPod, the iPhone, and the iPad, each with its own unique and helpful features, Apple created an entire array of products that consumers would easily identify with and someday demand. (Twenty years ago, who would have thought that a large majority of Americans would carry a phone or other multiuse electronic device in their pocket or purse?) And, Apple constantly updates its bevy of products with new must-have features. Steve Jobs's novel ideas were translated into a value proposition via a product line, which is now here to stay. This is in large part because Apple has successfully embraced and deployed each of Kahan's points.

How does one build a value proposition? Here are six tips from Lisa Furgison at Bplans, a popular website in California's Silicon Valley (2016):

- **Define your target audience:** Figure out who your customers are.

- **Know your competitors:** Define who are they and what services or products they offer.

- **Define the needs your product or business meets:** Explain how your product or service helps others.

- **Dispel myths:** Address inaccurate ideas about what your product or service may or may not be or do.

- **Create a clear mission and message:** Craft a message that connects with your brand and company image.

- **Bring it to life:** Find marketing channels to put your product or service out into the world.

 It is never too early to begin research for a new idea or business venture. The Internet offers virtually endless information on nearly any topic you can imagine. However, you must be able to sort opinion—which is quite often fictional—from fact. Information must come from sources that are accurate, verifiable, reliable, and credible.

Building a Brand

Branding is a marketing strategy that involves creating a differentiated name and image, often using a logo and/or tag lines, to make a positive impression with consumers and to attract and keep customers (Branding, n.d.). For example, the following tag lines attempt to convey the corresponding company's brand:

- **BMW:** "The ultimate driving machine"

- **Hilton:** "Stop clicking around"

- **Delta Airlines:** "The Delta difference"

- **Hertz Rental Cars:** "Let Hertz put you in the driver seat"

- **Dollar Shave Club:** "Our blades are fu**ing great"

Nurses have a dual role: to adequately represent both their own brand and their organization's brand. Both must reflect integrity, a commitment to excellence, and the delivery of quality health-related care or outcomes.

What Skills Are Needed to Potentiate Success?

According to Susan Packard (2015), a co-founder of HGTV, smarts, enthusiasm, and ambition will get you only so far. You must also acquire and demonstrate certain technical skills to become "conditioned" to advance in business.

What skills, exactly, are required? To find out, I asked a half-dozen nurse-leader colleagues one question: What are five things nurses should know about business and the business of healthcare? In general terms, here is what they said:

- **Finance:** This includes budget development and management (labor and supply); payment models for services driving change in healthcare; strategic plans; and margin estimates for organizational profit and loss.

- **Cost:** This includes the cost to do business; financial concepts relative to cost, time, and expenses (fixed, variable, productive, non-productive, worked, paid, controllable, and uncontrollable); what feasibility studies are; and what a "return on investment" exercise consists of.

- **Technology:** This includes understanding how to use technology for optimal tracking of information and decision-making.

- **Human resources:** This includes supply-and-demand economics; the impact of turnover; labor category shortage predictions; new and evolving professional roles; succession planning; labor management with collective bargaining (unionization); and recruitment and retention strategies across diverse age groups and gender.

- **Patient safety, quality improvement, and outcomes:** This includes determining how patient safety, quality improvement, and outcomes drive organizational change; and how resulting policy influences outcomes and metrics related to compensation for services rendered.

- **Business intelligence:** This includes using data to make a business case; using statistical process control to assess patterns in relevant data; using trends for risk analysis; and understanding predictive modeling.

- **Supply chain:** This refers to the process of acquisition through distribution and how it ties to the revenue cycle (order/purchase through payment).

- **Communication:** This refers to how inter- and intra-professional communication works (or doesn't) and how customer and organizational communication affect organizational culture and performance.

- **Business planning:** This could be for the growth of an existing service or to start a new line of business.

- **Capital budgeting (for equipment):** This refers to the processing and tracking of assets; useful life; how to build a case for new products; and so on.

- **The value of entrepreneurship:** This refers to how novel thinking translates to new and/or better results in human or system performance of an organization.

- **Innovation:** This includes applying radical and imaginative thinking to improve current systems and/or create new ones.

- **Culture:** This refers to ways to improve the work environment.

This list reads like an academic curriculum for management. Although some nurses may find the idea of a leadership role daunting and these topics uninteresting, they should be of interest to others—especially those interested in pursuing leadership in nursing and healthcare specialties.

In addition to the skills listed, it's worth noting that much success in business stems from leadership and decision-making—both deciding what to do and what *not* to do. Timing and good judgment are also key.

Skills obtained for technical expertise or "conditioning," as Packard (2015) explained, also help set a foundation from which to build. And experiences of all types add to your arsenal of weapons, which you can select for use when appropriate circumstances present themselves.

> *"The essence of strategy*
> *is choosing what not to do."*
> –Michael Porter

Finally, in business, it's imperative that you understand who your audience is. Fry (2015b) posits that more than one in three American workers are Millennials (ages 18 to 34). Indeed, at 75.4 million, Millennials have now surpassed Baby Boomers (74.9 million) as the largest living generation (Fry, 2015a). Mike Perlis (2016), a staff writer for *Forbes*, reported on a recent survey of a group of influential Millennials about what they want from their lives and work. According to the survey, 44% of respondents said their number-one financial priority was funding an entrepreneurial endeavor. Nearly 80% prefer urban living (in cities). Approximately 30% see no need to own a car, and 97% are optimistic about the future. They are very Internet- and social media savvy, having grown up with both. Clearly, this generation will change the face of business and drive the need for new opportunities.

This link from Pew Research shows the U.S. labor force by generation in 2015: http://www.pewresearch.org/fact-tank/2015/05/11/millennials-surpass-gen-xers-as-the-largest-generation-in-u-s-labor-force/.

To learn about the specifics of each generation relative to size and in comparison with others, see this link from Pew Research: http://www.pewresearch.org/fact-tank/2016/04/25/millennials-overtake-baby-boomers/.

GAMESMANSHIP IN BUSINESS

In her book *New Rules of the Game: 10 Strategies for Women in the Workplace* (2015), Susan Packard described her broad, strategic, and intentionally overarching approach to success in business as *gamesmanship.* This word is generally used to describe a scenario featuring competition, teammates, goals, competitors, and the need to practice a craft. In most types of games, there are winners and there are losers. Business is no different. In business, people are evaluated based on results, period. These results are reflected by myriad metrics, including financial information, customer-service scoring, outcomes specific to the type of service or business, and so on.

Conclusion

Big-picture opportunities in the healthcare industry in general and in nursing in particular are nearly endless. The world is changing at a record pace, and with that change come new opportunities for innovation. These opportunities enable savvy individuals to showcase their creativity, talent, and "preneurship," either inside or outside of formal organizations. The sky is the limit!

Keep an idea journal. Use it as a place where you can log ideas and further investigate those that have merit.

CONCEPT CAPTURE

To explore your interests in the business of nursing and/or healthcare, reflect on your answers to the following questions:

1. What are your interests? What are your strongest skills? What are you really passionate about?

2. Create an interest and skill inventory by thinking about what you really like to do and what you feel you are good at. To get you started, a nominally priced inventory (less than $10) can be found at this link: http://www.myplan.com/assess/interests.php. Then, match your results with relevant or new possibilities in the selected industry. The opportunities may be in an existing organization or one that is just starting.

3. If you are presently employed in an organization, are there opportunities for career learning and progression? (Sometimes the only way up is out.)

4. Do you know and understand your department, business unit, or organization's financial state of affairs?

5. What is your risk tolerance?

6. What do you know about finance?

7. Business is changing due to generational dynamics. Are you prepared to work with multiple generations in the future?

8. How tuned in are you to the needs of the future?

2

BUSINESS INFRASTRUCTURE

One often-overlooked business imperative is infrastructure. Business infrastructure forms a foundation from which a successful business can be built. It requires research, access to capital, use of standard business practices and work processes, and assistance from individuals with a variety of professional expertise.

Aspects of business infrastructure include the following:

- Business structure

- Obtaining startup capital

- Planning

- Putting together a team

- Following rules and regulations

- Obtaining professional expertise

- Tax-planning and record-keeping

- Managing risk

- Technology (acquisition and implementation)

This chapter covers each of these topics.

Types of Business Structures

Typically, one of the first tasks is to select the type of legal entity required to operate a business. Examples of types of business infrastructure include the following (U.S. Small Business Association, n.d.):

- **Sole proprietorship:** This is a basic business structure in which the owner is responsible for the assets and liability.

- **Partnership:** This business structure offers a variety of options, depending on the type of business and number of partners.

- **Corporation (C or S):** This business structure offers differing liability and tax protection depending on the size and scope of services or products offered.

- **Limited liability company (LLC):** This business structure is somewhat more flexible than a corporation, while limiting the liability of the owner(s).

- **Cooperative structure:** This business structure is designed to meet a need related to service or products via membership.

Depending on the nature of the business, each structure offers various advantages and potential disadvantages, particularly relating to legality and taxes.

ONLINE RESOURCES

For more information on business structures and other resources, see the following:

- **SBA: Starting & Managing (https://www.sba.gov/starting-business/choose-your-business-structure):** On this page, the U.S. Small Business Administration (SBA) offers advice about how to start a business and explicitly lists the pros and cons of each type of business structure.

- **IRS: Business Structures (https://www.irs.gov/businesses/small-businesses-self-employed/business-structures):** Visit this page, provided by the U.S. Internal Revenue Service (IRS), to explore business models, tax implications, and legal consequences of the various business structures.

- **IRS: A to Z Index for Business (https://www.irs.gov/businesses/small-businesses-self-employed/a-z-index-for-business):** Search for information about various business topics using the IRS's A to Z Index for Business. You can search by business type, subject, or area of specialty.

- **IRS: Operating a Business (https://www.irs.gov/businesses/small-businesses-self-employed/operating-a-business):** Find information about how to operate a business.

"Success usually comes to those who are too busy to be looking for it."
–Henry David Thoreau

Obtaining Startup Capital

Startup capital is required for almost any business. This capital may come from formal resources (bank loans, venture capital, angel or other investors) or from self-funding. Either way, obtaining capital is often among the most challenging parts of starting and/or being in business—a state made more frustrating by the fact that access to capital provides many more choices for entrepreneurs.

When obtaining a loan—regardless of the source—you must proceed with caution. Obtaining a loan is much more involved, time-consuming, and invasive than self-funding. Lenders will evaluate numerous financial and non-financial indicators, which may make it difficult for some to obtain funding for a new business idea. Depending on the level of capital resources necessary to get started, self-funding may be the only viable option.

Banks commonly favor those who have money (shown in bank accounts, investment statements, real estate holdings, and so on) and can show a track record of responsibility; conversely, they are extremely wary of those who don't. Funding decisions always involve an analysis of risk, with the knowledge that too much risk may result in no reward (hence, the trepidation around lending).

Planning

Successful businesses don't happen without planning. Anyone interested in owning a business must spend considerable time thinking through and writing three key types of plans:

- Strategic
- Business
- Marketing

All types of business planning require a learned set of skills from thorough research. Thoughtful consideration of unintended consequences, unexpected occurrences, and risk is imperative. Fortunately, many resources are available to facilitate proper planning on the path to success.

Your Strategic Plan

Your strategic plan will present the purpose and goals of the core business function(s). This plan is usually written in future tense and projects how the business will look over time. (Target timeframes are typically 1, 2, and 3 to 5 years in advance.) Essentially, your strategic plan is a roadmap of sequential steps: what will come first, what will come second, and what will keep your business "in business."

The key sections in a strategic plan are as follows:

- **Executive summary:** This is a one- or two-page summary of the strategic plan. This summary presents the business's mission, vision, and values; identifies goals; provides an overview of the process used to create the plan; outlines how the plan will be evaluated and at what frequency; and identifies who was involved in the development of the plan.

- **Company overview:** This section covers two key areas:

  - **Mission, vision, and values statements:** These are usually presented in short written statements or in a bulleted format.

  - **The company's history and achievements to date:** This might be longer (written in paragraph form). The idea here is to give readers a more comprehensive look at the company's past successes as well as toward future achievements. For startup companies with no history or achievements, this section should give a compelling vision of where the company wishes to be in the future.

- **Goals, strategies, and tactics:** This is the most important part of the strategic plan. It designates a roadmap for how the business will be operated and how performance will be measured. It should identify between three and five strategic goals supported by program, financial, administrative, and governance strategies.

- **Financial projections:** This section typically presents a 3-year picture of expected financial performance against stated budget expectations (typically called a *pro forma*). Data in this section are usually presented in tabular rows and columns (common to accounting and finance reporting) and will likely include the following categories:

  - **Revenue/sales forecast:** This is derived from services performed or products sold.

  - **Expenses:** This is the cost to perform services or create and deliver products.

  - **Projected profit (loss) with assumptions:** In other words, what profit does the company expect?

  - **Projected cash flow with assumptions:** This is a visual representation of what the company's expected cash will be and what it will be used for.

  - **Projected balance sheet:** This summarizes the assets, liabilities, and equity of the company.

  - **Financial ratios:** Common types of these include debt to equity (gross profit), price to earnings (liquidity), inventory turnover (time for products to move through the development to sales process), return on assets (profitability from assets), etc.

  - **Break-even analysis:** Can the business cover all of its expenses and make a profit?

- **Capital requirements:** What capital investment is required?

- **Sources of capital:** These might include self-funding, loans, investment from investors, etc.

- **Appendices:** This section, which is optional, should include additional documentation to support the plan's data. For example, if the business conducted a focus group to arrive at the mission, vision, and values statements, then an appendix might include a summary of the process and findings. Another common example might be a strengths, weaknesses, opportunities, threats (SWOT) analysis (including the internal and external environments).

ONLINE RESOURCES

For examples of how a strategic plan can be written and what to include, see the following resources:

- **United States Department of State Strategic Plan:** https://www.state.gov/documents/organization/223997.pdf

- **U.S. Department of Health and Human Services Strategic Plan:** https://www.hhs.gov/about/strategic-plan/index.html

- **Foundation Center 2020:** http://2020.foundationcenter.org/2011/01/

- **"Strategic Plan Template: What to Include in Yours" by Dave Lavinsky (2013c):** http://www.forbes.com/sites/davelavinsky/2013/10/18/strategic-plan-template-what-to-include/#478d448b47e1

Your Business Plan

The business plan identifies services or product offerings the business intends to sell. It outlines detailed operational strategies via the following:

- **Cover page:** This page includes the business name, address, and contact information (telephone numbers, standard mailing addresses, Internet site, web/electronic mail addresses, and so on).

- **Executive summary:** This section summarizes the most important points from the full business plan. If the business is new, a description of intentions, a timeline, and anticipated obstacles demonstrate a well-thought-out strategy for success. For an established business, the following information is ordinarily included:

  - **Accomplishments:** If the business is already established, this section should outline the key business objectives from the past and subsequent financial results to date to demonstrate successful performance. A new business would not have this information.

  - **Objectives:** This section states the major business objectives.

  - **Mission, vision, and values statements:** Include a brief description for each statement in this section.

  - **Performance metrics:** Conclude the executive summary with a statement about what the "keys to success" will be for this business.

Write the executive summary last. That way, you can better summarize the full business plan.

- **Company overview:** This is a brief and fact-based description of the business. It should include the following:

  - **What it does:** Describe what the company does or will provide to the marketplace; what will make it unique, competitive, and successful; what will make it attractive to potential customers; and its primary goals and objectives.

  - **Company ownership and legal entity:** Specify the chosen business structure and ownership (legal entity); describe the type of business (for example, manufacturing, merchandising, service, etc.); indicate licensing and permitting requirements; and include a brief history of the business (existing versus startup).

- **Location:** Note the location of the primary business with a setting description (indoor office, outdoors, virtual, and so on). (If you have not yet selected a location, note potential locations.) Also note why the location is beneficial along with its impact—such as how the location might help attract top talent and how it could draw customers (customer/traffic patterns, accessibility, etc.).

- **Products and services:** Indicate the type of problem the business is trying to solve or how the business will add value to an existing market. Also note how the product or service will be sold (direct, wholesale, via distributors, etc.) and include data to support future market growth. Finally, include a presentation of product and service offerings from the eyes of the customer to show value.

- **Suppliers:** Describe all suppliers or vendor partners in this section.

- **Customer service:** Outline strategies for working with customers before, during, and after a sale. Include competitive performance objectives and state how the company intends to listen to the "voice of the customer."

- **Manufacturing:** Include a description of the facility, specialized machinery, or equipment required to produce the product(s) and/or service.

- **Company leadership:** Prepare an organizational chart to depict the management structure for the business and describe the background and relevant professional experience of key leaders. Consider including resumes of the top team members (chief executive officer, chief financial officer, chief marketing executive, chief nursing executive, etc.) in an appendix.

- **Financial management:** Write and prepare this section using standard accounting and financial-planning methods. Ideally, a certified professional accountant or financial planner should prepare and/or review this section. Of critical importance is a solid explanation of business profitability. All startup and other relevant costs for the launch of the business must be clearly stated. A pro forma or detailed financial plan should be shown in an appendix of the business plan with key financial metrics displayed.

 For more on business planning, see Chapter 3, "Finance 101."

Your Marketing Plan

Chapter 5, "Marketing," offers a comprehensive explanation of the marketing process. However, a brief description is relevant for this section related to planning. A marketing plan describes who the target audience will be, how customers will be marketed to, and what sort of marketing approach will be used—for example, digital, mail, telephonic, electronic, etc. Having a full understanding of the competitive environment, potential customer base, and the types of products or services the business will offer are crucial to effective marketing.

Ideally, the strategy, business, and implementation plans should be aligned with the marketing plan.

Your Strategy and Implementation Plan

You can include the information discussed in this section in other plans (i.e., the business and/or marketing plans), or as a separate strategy and implementation plan. A suggested outline for a standalone strategy and implementation plan is as follows:

- **Marketing plan:** For more on developing your marketing plan, see Chapter 5.

- **Sales plan:** This plan outlines the following:

  - Sales objectives (short, medium, and long-term goals), resources required, and how they relate to the overall business plan

  - Resources required, such as employees, space needs, and equipment

  - Products or services to be sold

  - A sales activity analysis projected by team member

  - A training plan for the sales team

  - An analysis of sales strategy, or how the sales objectives will be achieved

- **Location and facilities:** This section notes where the business will be located and what type(s) of facilities will be used to produce the products and/or services. (This information may or may not be the same as that used in the business plan, depending on the timing of plan creation.)

- **Equipment and technology:** This section covers what type(s) of equipment and technological adjuncts may be required for the business.

- **Milestones:** This section describes measurable achievements indicating business performance.

- **KPIs:** See the following "Performance Metrics" sidebar.

PERFORMANCE METRICS

You should design performance metrics for each plan to measure predictions against actual operational performance. Performance metrics, such as key performance indicators (KPIs), are usually tracked at specific intervals. Intervals may differ based on the type of business; however, they are usually reported monthly, quarterly, year-to-date, year-to-year comparisons, and so on.

KPIs have the following characteristics:

- **Strategy:** KPIs represent the strategic objectives.

- **Targets:** KPIs measure actual performance against set targets. For most businesses, targets are defined in the budgeting process for the coming year. Targets must be measurable and may represent various forms of metrics (for example, achievement, reduction, absolute, zero, percentages, etc.).

- **Ranges:** Targets have ranges of performance—for example, above, met, or below target.

- **Color-coded ranges:** Ranges of performance are typically color-coded to give a quick visual of the overall performance. Common color-coded ranges are blue, which represents greater than 100% target achievement; green, which indicates the achievement of the target; yellow, which denotes that the median target has been achieved; and red, which indicates a below-target metric in need of improvement.

- **Timeframes:** Targets are assigned timeframes in which they are expected to be achieved. Common timeframes are monthly, quarterly, and annually.

- **Benchmarks:** Targets are measured against baseline performance, (previous period performance, an internal or external source, industry metrics, and so on.).

*"There are no secrets to success.
It is the result of preparation, hard
work and learning from failure."*
–Colin Powell

Putting a Team Together

Even the smallest businesses need a qualified team. Depending on the business type and size, initial team members may be assembled for startup only or for a more permanent arrangement. In either case, the owner(s) of the business should select a diverse group of people with complementary skills (Ellevate, 2013). Team members should have professional expertise, specific skills, competency, and knowledge of requisite business operations.

For more than 50 years, SCORE—a non-profit partner of the SBA—has been America's premier source of free and confidential small business advice for entrepreneurs and small businesses. There are more than 300 SCORE offices across the U.S., each offering free business mentoring and low- or no-cost workshops (SCORE Association, 2016). Visit their website for information on how to find a mentor or local chapter, and to find answers to basic business questions: https://www.score.org.

The business owner is typically the executive leader and is usually the responsible party for most business decisions. Other team members might include the following individuals:

- A project manager for a specific objective

- A business planner for growth projections

- A board of advisors

- Decision support from business analytics or analysts

- An information technologist for managing an intranet and other aspects of technology

- A panel of qualified mentors

For more on assembling your team, whether by insourcing or outsourcing, see Chapter 4, "Competency in Business."

> *"The way to get started is to quit talking and begin doing."*
> —*Walt Disney*

Rules, Regulations, and Obtaining Expertise

Almost all types of businesses require some type of registration, license, and/or permit to legally operate. For example, a consulting business entity often requires multiple types of licenses and/or registrations for federal and state compliance, such as registration with the Secretary of State (in each state where business is conducted), local and regional licenses to do business, tax entity registration, as well as professional licensure.

The SBA is an excellent resource for anyone starting or operating a small business, and its website has an entire section devoted to registering your business. Find it here: https://www.sba.gov/starting-business/choose-register-your-business.

To ensure you are compliant with rules and regulations, you will likely need to obtain expertise from outside sources. Outsourcing certain functions or tasks to the following types of professionals can also help you to be more productive. (You can find these professionals—who may themselves be small business owners—in almost every part of the country):

- **Bookkeeping:** A bookkeeper can help you maintain adequate business records.

- **Legal:** Legal professionals can offer you advice pertaining to contracting, law interpretation, copyright, trademarking, intellectual property protection, strategy, and legal compliance with existing business law.

- **Accounting:** Accountants have the expertise needed to ensure you meet accounting standards, and they can provide tax assistance related to planning and compliance with professional business standards.

- **Marketing:** Typical functions for marketing professionals include advertising, using social media, strategy planning for business growth, and more.

- **Technology:** These professionals can help you select and maintain computers, provide web design, and aid you in the planning of your inter- and intranet enterprise.

- **Clerical:** These professionals can assist you with tasks relating to organization, office management, errands, banking, and so on.

Tax-Planning and Record-Keeping

Tax-planning is the process of determining when, whether, and how to conduct business and personal transactions to reduce or eliminate tax liability. This aspect of business cannot be ignored, and should be viewed as an area of high risk.

The tax-reporting requirements of your business depend solely on its legal structure. Most businesses must file an annual federal income tax return or an informational return (partnerships). In addition to paying federal taxes, businesses must also pay taxes based on state, regional, and/or local law.

There are several types of federal taxes in the U.S.:

- **Income tax:** Federal income taxes are generally paid as income is earned by individuals and some types of businesses.

- **Self-employment tax:** Self-employed individuals must pay a self-employment tax, consisting of a combined rate set to fund social security (senior citizens, disability, and survivor benefits) and Medicare (health insurance).

- **Employment tax:** Businesses are required to pay employment taxes. These include social security, Medicare, individual federal income tax withholding, and federal unemployment (FUTA).

- **Excise tax:** This tax pertains to certain types of purchased goods (a common example is gasoline tax to fund road-related costs).

Depending on the state in which business is conducted, business owners may also be required to register to pay and/or collect sales tax. Common taxes applied to the sale of goods and services include the following:

- **Vendor tax:** A vendor tax is a tax paid by the business owner on the sale of goods and services.

- **Consumer tax:** The business owner collects this type of tax from consumers on behalf of the state.

- **Combination tax:** This tax is a combination of the vendor tax and the consumer tax. With this tax, the business owner pays a state-mandated vendor tax, but the cost for the tax is passed on to consumers.

- **Use tax:** A use tax may be imposed for the storage, use, or purchase of personal property that is not covered by sales tax—for example, leases, rentals, out-of-state automobile purchases, etc.

- **Business property tax:** This is a tax imposed on property used to conduct business.

- **Property tax:** Each state specifies law related to taxable property. Some states collect property tax from businesses via commercial real estate transactions.

State taxes may involve a graduated or a flat-rate method of taxation.

OBTAINING AN EMPLOYER IDENTIFICATION NUMBER

Most business entities must apply for a federal Employer Identification Number (EIN), which is required for tax purposes. To determine whether a business is required to obtain an EIN, review the following questions provided by the U.S. Internal Revenue Service (IRS, 2016). If the answer to any of these questions is yes, then an EIN is required.

- Do you have employees?
- Do you operate a business as a corporation or a partnership?
- Do you file any of these tax returns: employment, excise, alcohol, tobacco, and firearms?
- Do you withhold taxes on income, other than wages, paid to a non-resident alien?
- Do you have a Keogh plan?
- Are you involved with any of the following types of organizations?
  - Trusts (except certain grantor-owned revocable trusts), Individual Retirement Accounts (IRAs), exempt organization business income tax returns
  - Estates
  - Real estate mortgage investment conduits
  - Non-profit organizations
  - Farmers' cooperatives
  - Plan administrators

Read more about the EIN process and particulars here: https://www.irs.gov/businesses/small-businesses-self-employed/apply-for-an-employer-identification-number-ein-online.

Business owners are encouraged to clarify all tax laws with the appropriate entity when starting or running any type of business.

Business owners should be aware of common pitfalls related to business tax. These include (but are not limited to) the following:

- **Failure to report substantial amounts of income:** Examples include a shareholder's failure to report dividends, a store owner's failure to report portions of daily business receipts, undeposited income (cash), etc.

- **Claims for fictitious or improper deductions:** Examples include claiming excluded deductions, overstatement of expenses, excessive charitable contributions, etc.

- **Accounting irregularities:** Examples include the failure to keep adequate records, discrepancies discovered between financial records and corporate filings, etc.

- **Improper allocations of income:** Examples include contributions to children or a relative, gifting, donations, etc.

For these (and other) reasons, it is highly recommended that business owners engage a tax professional, such as a certified public accountant (CPA), to help with their taxes. A CPA will know of provisions for tax credits, deductions, and so on, of which the business owner might be unaware. They can also help the business owner complete tax-related forms.

In addition to assisting with tax-related issues, a tax professional may also provide bookkeeping services to ensure accurate recordkeeping. This is necessary for the completion of appropriate tax forms, licenses, and in preparation for auditing. Tax professionals can also provide general accounting services, such as reviewing the financial pro forma and/or financial statements for the business and recommending the best accounting method.

The most common accounting methods are cash and accrual. The cash method allows for the calculation of income and expenses in a single reporting period (typically annually). The accrual method allows for the reporting of income in the year it is earned and the deduction of expenses in the year they are incurred.

You can read more about the differences in accounting methods for various types of businesses here: http://www.inc.com/encyclopedia/accounting-methods.html.

ONLINE RESOURCES

There are a multitude of online resources for business owners to learn about taxation. Here are just a few recommended references:

- **IRS: Business Taxes:** https://www.irs.gov/businesses/small-businesses-self-employed/business-taxes

- **IRS: State Government Websites:** https://www.irs.gov/businesses/small-businesses-self-employed/state-links-1

- **SBA: Determine Your State Tax Obligations:** https://www.sba.gov/starting-business/filing-paying-taxes/determine-your-state-tax-obligations.

Risk Management

Starting a business is risky. Fortunately, there are ways to mitigate risk. Two of the best ways to mitigate risk are to purchase the proper insurance (to guard against mistakes) and to make sound business decisions based on data and industry norms. Both of these strategies deploy anticipatory thinking by being optimally prepared, and assist in building a defensible case should one end up in a court of law. Just as you have insurance to cover your home, your car, and your health, business owners must purchase insurance to cover their businesses—preferably *before* commencing operations.

Common types of business insurance—sometimes referred to as *business owner's insurance*—include the following (Newtek, 2012):

- **Professional liability insurance:** This covers a specific business or individual against negligence due to harm that results from a mistake or a failure to perform. It is commonly referred to as *errors and omissions (E&O) insurance.*

- **Property insurance:** This covers equipment, signage, inventory, and furniture in the event of a fire, storm, or theft. Mass-destruction events like floods and earthquakes are generally not covered under standard property insurance policies. (You may require a separate policy for expanded coverage.)

- **Director and officer insurance:** This protects the directors and officers of a corporation from claims related to their actions affecting the profitability and/or operations of a company.

- **Commercial or general liability insurance:** This covers a variety of types of claims for business owners—contractors, bodily injury, property damage, personal injury, and so on.

- **Worker's compensation insurance:** This covers medical treatment and provides disability and death benefits if an employee is injured or dies at work.

- **Unemployment insurance:** Programs of the Department of Labor are funded through unemployment insurance, which is collected through taxes. This insurance provides benefits to *eligible* workers who become unemployed.

- **Temporary disability insurance:** Businesses are required to pay this tax in California, Hawaii, New Jersey, Rhode Island, and Puerto Rico. This type of insurance is essentially income protection in the event of a disabling injury or illness. Many individuals also purchase this type of insurance for themselves (not employer sponsored).

- **Home-based business insurance:** Homeowner insurance policies generally do not provide adequate coverage for home-based businesses. Frequently, additional insurance or a rider is required for coverage of business equipment and inventory.

- **Product liability insurance:** This covers the business against liabilities related to products developed and sold.

- **Automobile insurance:** This covers vehicles used for business purposes. A variety of insurance options exist: third-party injury liability, occurrence, personal use, etc.

- **Business interruption insurance:** Should a disaster or catastrophic event occur that results in lost business days, business interruption insurance compensates the business for lost income during the interruption.

- **Life insurance:** This is for the company's protection in the event the business owner(s) dies.

- **Technology insurance:** This covers breaches of confidential or protected data/information.

It is highly recommended that all business owners fully investigate applicable insurance requirements. Brokers or insurance professionals can assist with the selection of appropriate coverage options. In addition, the SBA has information about insurance on its website at this address: https://www.sba.gov/managing-business/running-business/insurance/types-business-insurance.

Technology

Technology has changed and will continue to affect every part of the operation and management of business. Simply put, technology can benefit business owners by enhancing productivity, granting nearly immediate access to important information, and assisting in communication, not to mention the following areas:

- **Finance and marketing:** Digital and electronic methods have significantly affected these areas thanks to advances in computer science, networking, and communications technology.

- **The Internet:** The Internet has enabled small businesses to compete against much larger established firms in many operational areas. These include access, communications, advertising, customer-relation management, and social media.

- **Time management:** Technology has exponentially increased the speed of business. Business owners must engage with customers and manage their time as efficiently as possible by adopting relevant technology. Examples include the use of smartphones, face-to-face communication capabilities, Skype for online meetings with participants anywhere in the world, and so forth.

In today's world of big data and powerful analytics, the most striking transformation in the businesses of the future will relate to how they use technology to manage their relationships with and in the global marketplace. The greatest challenge for organizational leaders and business owners will be keeping up with the pace of technology-related change and reserving sufficient funding for capital technologic purchases.

Common Pitfalls

Often, new business owners quickly become overwhelmed and get caught up in the details of the business's day-to-day operations. Some common pitfalls include the following:

- Business owners fail to issue adequate direction or explicit instructions to others, resulting in objectives not being met.

- Leaders fail to ensure engagement by all team members, which often results in a lack of buy-in, lackadaisical focus, and shoddy execution of planning objectives, which negatively affects the project budget, schedule, and deliverables.

- Too much attention is paid to data collection, and not enough to data analysis and strategic insight. Often, team members like to deal with "what ifs." However, this is usually a waste of time. Decisions must be objective and based solely on data.

- Strategic thinking is mistaken for strategic planning. Thinking strategically about something does not typically result in action toward obtaining a result. Strategic planning, on the other hand, involves designing a series of activities to be executed to move toward a goal.

- Teams rush to implement the first strategy that satisfies the majority of team members. Instead, teams should use a decision-making algorithm for effective prioritization, to assess the effort required, and to estimate the overall impact of decisions.

It is critical to stay focused and keep sight of the big picture—that is, the original objectives outlined in the strategic, business, and marketing plans. To achieve success, business owners must balance the daily details with big-picture thinking.

EXERCISE

What are some strategies you could use to mitigate—if not avoid altogether—the common pitfalls identified in this section?

1. _____

2. _____

3. _____

What other pitfalls might arise?

1. _____

2. _____

3. _____

Conclusion

Outlining the proper steps to create and/or run a business is critical to a successful outcome. Business infrastructure requires careful thought, thorough research, and action toward big-picture goals. Each of the sections in this chapter are of equal importance: business structure, capital acquisition, planning, adequate measurement, team selection, managing risk, using technology, and following standard rules. While business can be somewhat complicated, it can also be a gratifying adventure!

CONCEPT CAPTURE

To begin building an adequate business infrastructure, reflect on the following questions:

1. What type of business structure will meet the needs of the business?

2. Is enough capital available/reserved for infrastructure?

3. What type of professional assistance might you need to begin the planning process?

4. What KPIs would demonstrate business success?

5. Who should be on the business owner's team?

6. What risk-management strategies will the business use?

7. What type(s) of insurance is required?

8. What type of equipment, technology, and/or supplies will the business need to conduct business?

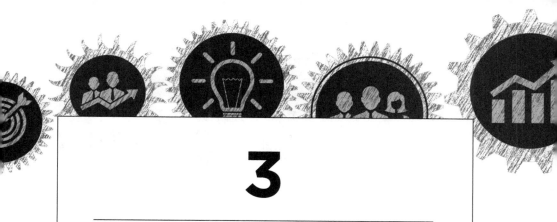

3

FINANCE 101

Business success requires "financial fitness." You must understand basic financial concepts and their application, and be able to converse intelligently with those who possess financial expertise.

Finance makes the world turn. Inflows and outflows keep the global economy moving. Finance is related to nearly every aspect of business: start-up, daily operations, and planning for the future. This chapter aims to give you a basic understanding of how finance works in the world of business.

If you're not well-versed on the terminology used in this chapter, see Appendix A, "Basic Financial Definitions." It provides a glossary of common financial terms.

> *"A good financial plan is a road map that shows us exactly how the choices we make today will affect our future."*
> –Alexa Von Tobel

Types of Financial Statements

There are three basic financial statements. These are as follows (Financial statement, n.d.; *Inc.*, n.d.):

- **Balance sheet:** This statement shows a firm's assets, liabilities, and net worth on a stated date.

- **Income statement:** Also called *profit and loss accounting*, this statement shows how the net income is derived in a stated period.

- **Cash-flow statement:** This statement shows the inflows and outflows of cash caused by a firm's activities during a stated period.

Balance Sheet

Typical items on a balance sheet (see Figure 3.1) consist of the following (Waddill-Goad, 2015):

- **Assets**

  - Cash and investments

  - Accounts receivable (AR), measured in days

- Materials/inventory/consumables in stock (the supply chain's current assets)

- Fixed assets (machinery and equipment)

- Real property (real estate)

- Work in progress (manufacturing)

- Finished goods (products)

- **Liabilities**

  - Loans (short- or long-term)

  - Taxes (due)

- **Equity**

  - Beginning balance

  - Profit/loss (the cycle for the current year)

Income Statement

Typical items on an income statement (see Figure 3.2) consist of the following (Waddill-Goad, 2015):

- **Sales or revenue:** Income from goods sold or services rendered

- **Cost of goods sold:** A delineation of the cost of labor versus materials

- **Contribution margin:** Common costs such as overhead, depreciation, unsold capacity, etc.

- **Operating expenses:** Costs associated with doing business (producing a product or service)

  - **Operating margin:** Revenue left after paying variable expenses (see the categories in Figure 3.2)

  - **Net income (the bottom line):** Net profit or loss

	Current Year	Prior Year	Change
ASSETS			
Current Assets			
Cash	$49,200	$92,000	-$42,800
Accounts Receivable	$17,000	$15,120	$1,880
Inventory	$163,500	$112,480	$51,020
Total Current Assets	$229,700	$219,600	$10,100
Other Assets			
Equipment	$56,000	$42,000	$14,000
Land and Buildings	$650,000	$650,000	$0
Automotive Vehicles	$70,000	$70,000	$0
Total Other Assets	$776,000	$762,000	$14,000
TOTAL ASSETS	$1,005,700	$981,600	$24,100
LIABILITIES			
Current Liabilities			
Accounts Payable	$25,000	$9,800	$15,200
Current Portion of Loans	$23,750	$23,750	$0
Bank Overdraft	$8,000	$0	$8,000
Line of Credit	$6,750	$11,650	-$4,900
Tax Liability	$30,000	$23,000	$7,000
Total Current Liabilities	$93,500	$68,200	$25,300
Non-Current Liabilities			
Long-Term Business Loan (Startup)	$356,250	$393,750	-$37,500
Long-Term Business Loan 2 (Expansion)	$45,000	$55,000	-$10,000
Total Non-Current Liabilities	$401,250	$448,750	-$47,500
TOTAL LIABILITIES	$494,750	$516,950	-$22,200
EQUITY			
Owners' Equity	$491,850	$455,700	$36,150
Current Year Income (Loss)	$19,100	$8,950	$10,150
Total Equity	$510,950	$464,650	$46,300
TOTAL LIABILITIES & EQUITY	$1,005,700	$981,600	$24,100

Figure 3.1   An example of a balance sheet.

REVENUE/INCOME			PERCENT OF REVENUE
	Merchandise Sales	$312,000	
	Other Income	$12,750	
	Total Revenue	$324,750	
COST OF GOODS SOLD			
	Direct Labor	$129,832	
	Direct Materials	$86,918	
	Total Cost of Goods Sold	$216,750	
CONTRIBUTION MARGIN		$108,000	33.26%
OPERATING EXPENSES			
	Wages and Benefits	$68,000	
	Misc. Supplies	$1,500	
	Rent and Utilities	$5,400	
	Total Operating Expenses	$74,900	
OPERATING MARGIN		$33,100	10.19%
NON-OPERATING EXPENSES			
	Depreciation Expense	$9,000	
	Rental Expense	$4,500	
	Interest Expense	$500	
	Total Non-Operating Expenses	$14,000	
NET INCOME/(LOSS)		$19,100	5.88%

Figure 3.2   An example of an income statement.

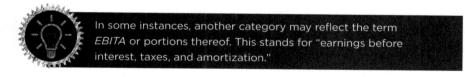

In some instances, another category may reflect the term *EBITA* or portions thereof. This stands for "earnings before interest, taxes, and amortization."

Cash-Flow Statement

The management of cash flow in any type of business is essential. The cash flow of a business reflects how likely it is the business will be able to pay its outstanding liabilities (bills).

A standard cash-flow statement simply shows the flow of money (cash) in and out of a business. This statement is "pure"—that is, it shows a true picture of a business. This is in contrast to other types of statements, which could reflect accounting nuances and may be a bit more difficult to interpret.

> *"Rule No. 1: Never lose money.*
> *Rule No. 2: Never forget Rule No. 1."*
> *–Warren Buffet*

In 1987, the Financial Accounting Standards Board (FASB) issued a "Statement of Financial Accounting Standards," which required businesses to issue a financial statement of cash flow rather than a statement of changes in financial position (*Inc.*, n.d.).

Typical items on a cash-flow statement (see Figure 3.3) consist of the following (*Inc.*, n.d.; Waddill-Goad, 2015):

- **Cash from operations:** This is cash generated from the day-to-day operations of the business.

- **Cash from investments:** This is cash used for investing as well as cash obtained from the sale of assets. Assets may include business equipment or other businesses within a corporate structure.

- **Cash from financing:** This includes cash paid or issued through the borrowing of money from another entity. For example, with a start-up business, the cash needed to begin operation commonly comes from the owner(s) or from a business loan. Money from owners is shown as equity on the balance sheet, whereas a business loan is reflected as a long-term liability (debt).

- **Net increase or decrease in cash:** This includes cash compared to previous periods (such as other months, quarters, or years).

The website of the Small Business Association (SBA) offers more information about cash flow and numerous other useful resources for small businesses. You can find them here: https://www.sba.gov/blogs/projecting-your-business-cash-flow-made-simple?leavingSBA=.

CASH FLOW FROM OPERATING ACTIVITIES		
Net Income	$19,100	
Adjustments to Reconcile Net Income to Net Cash		
Provided by Operating Activities:		
Depreciation on Fixed assets	$9,000*	$28,100
(Increase) Decrease in Current Assets:		
Accounts Receivable	($1,880)	
Inventory	($51,020)	
Prepaid Expenses	$0	($52,900)
Increase (Decrease) in Current Liabilities:		
Accounts Payable	$15,200	
Accrued Expenses and Unearned Revenues	$0	$15,200
NET CASH PROVIDED (USED)		**($9,600)**
CASH FLOW FROM INVESTING ACTIVITIES		
Purchase of Equipment	($14,000)	
Purchase of Real Property	$0	
NET CASH PROVIDED (USED)		**($14,000)**
CASH FLOW FROM FINANCING ACTIVITIES		
Proceeds from Line of Credit	$0	
Payments on Line of Credit	($4,900)	
Proceeds from Long-Term Debt	$0	
Payments on Long-Term Debt	($47,500)	
NET CASH PROVIDED (USED)		**($52,400)**
NET INCREASE (DECREASE) IN CASH	($42,800)	
BEGINNING CASH BALANCE	$92,000	
NET INCREASE (DECREASE) IN CASH	($42,800)	
ENDING CASH BALANCE		**$49,200**
*Tax Liability and Depreciation are Non-Cash Expenses		
ACTUAL BALANCE SHEET CASH BALANCE **(Shown in Figure 3.1)**		**$49,200**

Figure 3.3 An example of a cash-flow statement.

SCORE, a small-business support organization, offers a gallery of free templates for business planning, financial statements, marketing, sales, and management on its website. You can find these templates here: https://www.score.org/resource/business-planning-financial-statements-template-gallery.

"At base, financial literacy is inextricably connected to control over one's future."
–Ann Cotton

Reviewing Financial Statements

When reviewing financial statements, consider the following questions:

- **What are the key success factors for the organization to achieve maximum profitability?** Businesses are profitable when expenses are monitored and maintained within expected budget projections. Expenses such as labor and supplies (which represent the two largest expenses for most businesses) require close monitoring and adjustment when operating outside of expected budget projections. A successful business leader focuses equally on both expenses and profitability.

- **How is the organization's financial performance?** All business leaders have some idea of the profit margin they expect to achieve in operating their business. This profit margin depends on the type of business. In healthcare, a profit margin of 3% or more is considered good, and profit margins greater than 5% are considered excellent (Kutscher, 2014; The Economist, 2010). When profit margins fail to meet expectations, business leaders must identify opportunities for improvement by examining every aspect of the business. When opportunities for improvement are identified, the business owner must take corrective action.

- **What is the profit (or loss) for each major payer or product line?** If the business sells services to more than one type of payer (for example, contractual, fee for service, cash, charity, etc.) or offers more than one service in a business, the business owner must evaluate the profitability of each one, from the standpoint of both payer revenue and individual service profitability. Depending on the business model, the business might offer services under a contractual basis, charging a specific rate for a specified payer. Or, the business might choose to charge a fee-for-service for each service provided. For example, if you run a business for which an insurance company is the payer, payment for services rendered might be a requirement of the contractual arrangement. If the arrangement is a fee-for-service, the business would set the fee for the service and collect payment accordingly. In some cases, a business might allow the acceptance of cash or provide a charitable service. In these cases, the business must follow standardized accounting principles to record all business transactions. If not all the products or services offered are profitable, ongoing evaluation will show whether they should remain as a core business offering, be scaled back, or be discontinued altogether. Remember: No margin, no mission!

"Financial literacy is an issue that should command our attention because many Americans are not adequately organizing finances for their education, healthcare, and retirement."
–Ron Lewis

Access to Capital

The success of any business depends on adequate access to different types of capital throughout the business's start-up and growth cycle. Some business owners rely on debt and equity financing to start and expand or grow businesses, as well as to support fundamental business functions such as marketing, manufacturing, and sales. These sources of funding can also support research and development (R&D) and innovation.

During the early stages of a business start-up, many business owners experience negative cash flow. This is often a result of poor planning and because they underestimate how much capital the business will need. Indeed, most new businesses fail (80%) within the first 18 months because they simply run out of cash (Wagner, 2013). Other reasons cited for small-business failure include the following (Thorpe, 2014):

- Failure to market online
- Failure to listen to customers
- Failure to leverage growth opportunities
- Failure to adapt when the market changes
- Inadequate tracking and measuring of marketing efforts

Before asking for a business loan, all business owner(s) must prepare. Here are some points to consider before contacting a lender:

- **Is the business owner (you) "loan application ready"?** Has your personal credit score (called a *FICO score*) been evaluated, and is it high enough to qualify for a loan? FICO scores range from 300 to 850, with higher values indicating higher levels of credit trustworthiness. Ninety of the one hundred largest U.S. lending institutions use FICO scores to make consumer credit decisions (Fair Isaac Corporation, n.d.). Lenders typically require a FICO score of at least 670. A score above 740 is good, and one above 800 is exceptional (Experian Information Services, Inc., 2015). You can check your FICO score at the following reputable credit agency websites:
- **Experian:** http://www.experian.com
- **TransUnion:** https://www.transunion.com
- **Equifax:** http://www.equifax.com

FICO SCORES

FICO scores influence the amount of credit a lender is willing to loan and the rate of interest for repayment. An individual's FICO score is calculated based on the following factors (Experian Information Solutions, Inc., n.d.):

- Credit payment history (35%)
- Outstanding credit debt (30%)
- Length of time the individual has had a line of credit (15%)
- New credit activity (10%)
- The types of credit used (10%)

Low FICO scores are typically associated with a history of unpaid bills, past due or defaults of loan payments, tax liens, and so on.

- **Do you have sources of income outside the business sufficient to cover your monthly living expenses?** During the information-gathering and analysis process, lenders look for a stable income history and a strong credit rating. Be prepared to disclose previous years of income-tax returns, bank statements, investment account statements, and employment history, as well as any pertinent sources of income or debt such as retirement, disability, child support, alimony, etc.

The SBA has an excellent example of a personal financial statement, which can also be used as a business-assessment tool. You can find it here: https://www.sba.gov/sites/default/files/forms/SBA_Form_413_7a-504-SBG.pdf.

- **Is the business plan well-designed and well-written?** Typically, no lender will grant funding to a business owner unless a solid business plan is in place. This business plan should contain a general description of the business, a budget, a description of funding needs, projections for the first two or three years (again, this is called a *pro forma*), and how market research supports the business plan's projections. In addition, lenders will want to evaluate market competition and the business's likelihood of success.

When writing the business plan, consider using Business Plan Pro, which is widely considered the best business-planning software. For information about the software, visit http://www.businessplanpro.com/template_offer_lt2/.

- **Does your resume reflect your ability to run the business successfully?** A resume is an important document that conveys your educational and professional background as well as your business readiness. Highlighting business skills, accomplishments, and experiences (specifically tied to the business plan) will solidify your prospects for approval.

- **Do you have sufficient collateral to ensure a capital investment?** Most lenders require some level of collateral to cover a stated percentage of the loan value. For very high-risk businesses, collateral may go as high as 100% of the loan value. Very few lenders offer loan options that do not involve collateral.

Read more about loan collateral on the SBA's website: https://www.sba.gov/loans-grants/get-ready-apply/check-your-credit/collateral.

Lenders make decisions based on how informed and prepared you, the business owner, are. To demonstrate your level of preparedness, ask the lender these questions during your first meeting:

- What is the interest rate for the loan?

- Will the interest rate be fixed or variable?

- Will there be a requirement for insurance? If so, what kind of insurance will be required? (Types of insurance could be life, liability, property, flood, directors and officers, and so on.)

- Will there be a monthly service fee for the loan? If so, how much is the fee and what services are included?

- If you have other accounts with the lending institution, are discounts on the loan interest rate available?

- Is there a loan fee to obtain the loan? If so, what is the fee?

- Is there a penalty for early payment? If so, what is the penalty?

- Does the lender offer any value-added services after loan activation that might assist a new business owner—for example, business training, education, or workshops?

Business owners should thoroughly investigate available options for accessing capital. These include both private and public funding sources:

- **Private funding sources:** Private investment firms may offer private equity (PE), venture capital (VC), and/or angel investing (AI). Read more about private investment here: https://www.sba.gov/blogs/how-find-right-private-investor-your-small-business-0.

- **Public funding sources:** The public sector can play a facilitating role by offering tax credits and providing funding to innovative companies to cover some start-up costs. The goal of public-sector investment is to stimulate private investment in a business or businesses. After all, the formation of a new business in the community may create new jobs. In addition, cash generated by the company will likely flow through the local economy.

In addition, due to the growth of the Internet and social networking, there are two new funding options to consider:

- **Crowdfunding:** This generates start-up funds through monetary contributions by numerous investors via the Internet in exchange for early access to the initial product or for firm equity.

Examples of crowdfunding websites include the following:

- **Fundable (for start-ups):** http://www.fundable.com/

- **RepayVets (for veterans):** https://www.facebook.com/ RepayVets/

- **GoFundMe (for anything):** https://www.gofundme.com/

- **LendingClub (for anything):** https://www.lendingclub. com/

- **Kickstarter (for anything):** https://www.kickstarter.com/ about?ref=nav

The North American Securities Administrators Association (NASAA) website contains information about intrastate crowdfunding opportunities: http://www.nasaa.org/ industry-resources/corporation-finance/instrastate-crowdfunding-resource-center/intrastate-crowdfunding-directory/.

- **Peer-to-peer:** This electronic platform for business lenders takes advantage of big data-processing capabilities to rapidly assess firm risk and serve as a broker for small-business loans.

After the business acquires capital, funds must be used according to the business plan and its budget. Close monitoring of revenue and expenses is crucial. The ability to make timely adjustments to achieve budget targets is of the utmost importance. All loan payments must be paid on time and in full. The inability of the business to make monthly debt payments is a strong signal to the lender that their investment may be at risk. Business owners are encouraged to keep open lines of communication with their lending institution(s) and loan officer and to work with both if any issues arise regarding repayment.

> *"In the business world,*
> *the rearview mirror is always*
> *clearer than the windshield."*
> —*Warren Buffet*

Start-up Considerations and Business Analysis

Merriam-Webster (Start-up, n.d.,-b) defines a start-up as "the act or an instance of setting in operation or motion" or "a fledging business enterprise." The American Heritage Dictionary Online (Start-up, n.d.,-a) defines start-up as "a business or undertaking that has recently begun operation."

Both new businesses (that is, start-ups) and businesses that offer new services require *all* the business owner's time and attention to get off the ground. Many start-ups fail due to both inadequate planning and a lack of focus by the business owner related to finance, business development, and leadership.

Ryan Allis, previous chief executive officer (CEO) of a start-up business in the San Francisco, California Bay Area called iContact, wrote *The Startup Guide* (http://startupguide.com/entrepreneurship/introduction/) to assist others in their journey as entrepreneurs. In it, he describes the trials and tribulations that he and his business partner faced on their path to success.

Each department, division, or service line in any business entity should be viewed as a smaller business within a business. The following structure has been developed for a business or unit analysis by Suzanne M. Waddill-Goad & Company, Inc. and has been used with permission. This structure of analysis has been refined over nearly two decades to obtain a snapshot of a variety of types of healthcare enterprises.

It uses a balanced scorecard approach with the typical pillars found in today's business operations.

- **Pillar 1: Finance**
  - Budget
  - Position control
  - Scheduling practices
  - Labor expenses
  - Non-labor expenses
  - Capital planning
  - Asset tracking
- **Pillar 2: Quality**
  - Regulatory compliance (accrediting or licensing bodies and industry standards)
  - Compliance (comparison with national or local metrics, clinical and non-clinical)
  - Defects (unexpected occurrences and risk analysis)
  - Culture of safety
  - High reliability
- **Pillar 3: People**
  - Recruitment and retention initiatives
  - Competency assessment
  - Job description structure
  - Training, education, and development programs
  - Leadership (qualified and effective)
  - Succession planning
  - Organizational structure

- **Pillar 4: Service**

  - Customer value and satisfaction (all groups of stakeholders)

  - Employee engagement

  - Service provider recruitment and retention

  - Human resource metrics (turnover, leaves of absence, scheduled and unscheduled absenteeism, etc.)

  - Work environment (culture)

- **Pillar 5: Growth**

  - Strategic plans (marketing, business, etc.)

  - Brand recognition

  - Advertising

  - Growth strategies (based on market and competition)

Records of Business Activity

All businesses must develop standard procedures for bookkeeping, accounting, and financial reporting. Financial procedures for optimal industry compliance should follow federal, state, and local laws. Using best practices is essential to being on the cutting edge in your business or industry.

There are multiple record-keeping systems available for purchase. In addition, most successful business owners seek accounting and legal advice from licensed professionals. Credible licensed accounting and legal professionals are knowledgeable about the abundant requirements, changing regulations, and standard practices that apply to most types of businesses.

Businesses should create and maintain the following records:

- **Contractual templates:** These precisely describe the scope of work to be performed. These provide both the business owner and the client an opportunity to clarify the services to be provided before work actually begins. Typical contracts exist for these common types of business arrangements:

  - Service contracts for independent contractors or companies

  - Product contracts for vendors or suppliers

  - Employment contracts, typically used to pay high-level or temporary employees

- **Accounting and tax records:** Accurate accounting and tax records assist owners in financial analyses and help determine the profitability of the business. For most businesses, the following records are required:

  - Business expenses

  - Credit-card statements

  - Bank statements

  - Annual tax returns

  - Quarterly tax filings and/or payment history

  - Payroll statements

  - Inventory

  - Sales

  - Income

  - Petty cash

  - Vehicle use log

  - Travel log

- Cash-register receipts

- Credit-card sales receipts

- Invoices

- Canceled checks and/or check stubs

- **Other records:** These depend on the type of business and may include the following:

  - Purchase orders

  - Employment applications

  - Electronic mail (email) and other business communications

  - Personnel records

  - Accident reports

  - Legal documents (such as documents outlining the Articles of Incorporation)

  - Permits (business or building)

  - Licenses (business or professional)

  - Intellectual property (such as trademark and service registrations and patents)

Compliance, which is a comprehensive effort to ensure businesses and their employees conduct operations and activities in an ethical manner, is another area that requires careful record-keeping. All business should be conducted with the highest level of integrity and in compliance with legal and regulatory requirements. Reasons for developing a compliance program might include the following:

- To develop a culture of ethics and compliance that is central to all operations and activities of the business

- To develop an understanding of the nature of risk and potential areas of exposure

- To identify and manage risk that may affect the operations and reputation of the business

- To integrate the compliance program into a business risk mitigation framework

Ideally, ethics and compliance programs should be designed to reflect the unique components of the business's specific operations. These programs should be based on the standard elements of an effective compliance program. For healthcare entities, the Office of Inspector General (OIG) provides compliance-related suggestions in a series of helpful documents, found here: https://oig.hhs.gov/compliance/compliance-guidance/index.asp.

The OIG also lists the seven major components of an effective ethics and compliance program, which can be found here: https://oig.hhs.gov/authorities/docs/cpgnf.pdf. They are as follows (OIG, 2000):

- High-level oversight should be provided by a chief compliance officer (CCO), who reports directly to the business's board of directors. For smaller businesses, a legal representative(s) may fulfill this function.

- Written standards and policies should be available for employees to follow and for external agencies to review (when appropriate).

- Training for all employees should include an initial and annual ethics and compliance training module. Depending on the type of business, consideration should be given to extending this training to selected high-risk contractual entities.

- Auditing and monitoring should include an annual risk assessment with appropriate development of a correction plan for substandard findings.

- There should be open lines of communication through various methods, including an anonymous reporting system, easy-to-use employee reporting, external auditing, and internal audit results.

- Response to detected deficiencies (which should be described in the corrective action plan) should include the following elements:

  - Identification of the issue

  - Revisions to policies and procedures, if necessary

  - Training related to new or revised policies and procedures

  - Monitoring to ensure compliance

  - Appropriate disciplinary action for employees in the event of non-compliance

- Disciplinary action (as warranted) must be delivered by leadership when employees, contractors, or others who are to abide by the ethics and compliance program intentionally violate its standards. Corrective action should be levied based on severity and may include termination of employment.

"If you create incredible value and information for others that can change their lives—and you always stay focused on that service— the financial success will follow."
–Brendon Burchard

When businesses fail to follow an established ethics and compliance program, and to take action when necessary, it indicates that leadership has lost its focus and commitment to being credible to employees, business partners, and, in some instances, the communities in which they operate. Leaders who demonstrate ethical leadership are necessary to provide a moral compass for employees and to set a comprehensive culture of compliance for the business.

Revenue Cycles and Financial Planning

The primary objective of conducting a revenue cycle review is to secure optimal reimbursement from payers. This review may also uncover opportunities for improvement in financial performance to ensure long-term viability. Businesses must design systems to capture all available revenue. Strategies to meet that goal include the following:

- **Informing clients that payment is expected at the time of service or an agreed-upon timeframe (for example, within 30, 60, or 90 days):** At the first point of contact, finance staff should begin a dialogue with the client regarding the collection of copay or co-insurance, with outstanding balances regularly tracked and reported.

- **Effectively communicating with clients:** The financial team must gather accurate demographic information, convey payment responsibilities, and pursue collections when necessary.

- **Removing barriers for easy payment:** Leveraging technology for revenue tracking and online payment is essential.

- **Reducing the number of late arrivals and no-shows:** This means implementing a comprehensive policy and automated electronic appointment reminders.

- **Verifying registration information and insurance eligibility:** This eliminates the odds of providing services that are not covered and of being denied payment.

- **Avoiding claim-submission errors due to inaccuracy:** An accurate electronic claim-submission process normally shortens payment turnaround time.

The American Medical Association (AMA) offers a bevy of resources for processing claims on its website: https://www.ama-assn.org/practice-management/managing-patient-payments.

- **Monitoring and managing non-payment for services rendered:** Businesses should have policies and procedures to deal with late payments, rejections, denials, and outstanding receivables. Revenue-cycle reviews should include the identification of outliers, common payment patterns, and root causes for problem areas.

- **Tracking charity services and account write-offs:** These should be tracked for future analysis.

The Healthcare Financial Management Association (HFMA) offers an excellent resource on strategies for a high-performance revenue cycle. You can find it here: http://www.hfma.org/Content.aspx?id=1729.

Effective revenue-cycle practices help business owners achieve tighter control over service eligibility, payer verification, and claims processing, and minimize denials of payment. Questions business owners may want to consider when reviewing monthly financial statements include the following:

- Are the accounts receivables aging at the planned rate (being paid in a timely manner and as projected)?

- Are too many accounts aging past the expected payment goal?

- What are the claim- and payment-rejection rates?

- Are there any troubling trends?

- What is the collection rate on billed charges?

- Are any point-of-service collections being missed?

- How many accounts are or need to be sent to a collection agency?

Reviewing these questions during monthly financial overviews can help you identify potential problems with payment claims, payments received, and payments needing to be collected.

 Business owners must incorporate sound financial management—in both theory and concept—to aid their managerial and personal decision-making. This includes developing skills to judge the validity of analyses performed by others, such as financial staff or consultants.

Each year, businesses should identify specific revenue-cycle performance measures and regularly track them against performance. These performance indicators might include the following:

- Revenue and expenses

- Charges (gross and net collection)

- Payments and adjustments to payments

- A comparison between averages and historical data (to assess whether the organization regularly receives full and timely payment for services rendered)

- Accounts receivable aging by payer (to gauge the timeliness of payment)

Business owners must measure key metrics and implement course-correction when required. This process of the revenue-cycle and financial-performance reviews is nearly continuous.

It's much easier to monitor key metrics using a dashboard that visually depicts the essential targets. Lavinsky (2013a) describes the importance of executive dashboards and shows a number of examples here: https://www.forbes.com/sites/davelavinsky/2013/09/06/executive-dashboards-what-they-are-why-every-business-needs-one/#75323efa37d1.

Managing Expenses for a Return on Investment

Successful business owners closely manage business expenses and are quick to make corrections if expenses exceed revenue projections. Expenses must be itemized and are typically displayed in a chart of accounts that groups like expenses into categories for tracking and trend comparison. General categories include the following:

- **Start-up costs:** These include all the costs of opening a business.

- **One-time costs:** These include capital expenditures such as incorporation fees, costs associated with securing real estate, trademark or registration application fees, initial inventory, vehicles, licenses, permits, etc.

- **Ongoing costs:** These include rent, utilities, office supplies, insurance, employee wages, actual expenses related to conducting business, and so on. Costs in this category typically align with the profit and loss statement.

- **Necessary expenses:** These include items that the business cannot do without, such as business licenses, insurance, etc.

- **Optional expenses:** These are items the business could operate without or could operate with via minimal cost. Examples include the use of shared office space versus traditional rent in a single office space, labor expenses versus the owner(s) doing all the various types of work (no cost), and so on.

Managing business expenses and keeping costs down is important for every new business owner and for all businesses as they continue to grow. Growth must be effectively balanced with managing the day-to-day operational needs. Maintaining this balance lessens the chances of the business increasing costs without compensatory growth. Many businesses face failure if expenses outpace revenue.

Figure 3.4 shows a chart of accounts, Figure 3.5 shows a trial balance, and Figure 3.6 shows a profit and loss statement. Each of these is important to the business. The chart of accounts outlines types of categories or accounts (relating to the overall financial picture) in the general ledger of the business. A trial balance is an accounting (or bookkeeping) report that shows the general ledger's accounts and monetary balances for a business at a specific point in time. The balances will either be a credit balance (income) or a debit balance (expenses and/or losses).

Account	Type
102 Checking	Bank
105 Accounts Receivable	AR
107 Funds from Stockholder	Current Asset
109 Retainers	Current Asset
110 Furniture and Fixtures	Current Asset
201 Accounts Payable	AP
206 Loan from Sole Proprietor	Current Liability
207 Loan from Owner	Current Liability
208 Payroll	Current Liability
260 Retained Earnings	Equity
300 Consulting Income	Income
312 Book Income	Income
401 Bank Service Charges	Expense
404 Memberships and Affiliations	Expense
406 Postage	Expense
408 Dues and Subscriptions	Expense

Figure 3.4   An example of a chart of accounts.

Balance Sheet Accounts:	
Assets	$1,005,700
Liabilities	($494,750)
Owner's (Stockholder's) Equity	($510,950)
Income Statement Accounts:	
Operating Revenues	($324,750)
Cost of Goods Sold	$216,750
Operating Expenses	$74,900
Non-Operating Expenses	$14,000
Net Income (Loss)	($19,100)

Figure 3.5   An example of a trial balance.

Revenue	($324,750)
Cost of Goods Sold	$216,750
Gross Margin	**($108,000)**
Operating Expenses	$74,900
Income from Operations	**($33,100)**
Other Income and Expenses	$14,000
Net Income	**($19,100)**

Figure 3.6   An example of a profit and loss statement.

*"Business requires understanding
financial matters, but management
is different from running the financial
aspects of the business—it requires
understanding complex systems,
how they operate, the nature of
organisations, what happens when
people interact in groups, and
how to motivate and guide people."*
–Elizabeth Moss Kanter

Nuances in Healthcare Finance

The U.S. healthcare industry is unique in several key ways. First, it is composed of two main types of businesses, each with its own business model:

- **Not-for-profit (NFP) organizations:** These are run privately or by the government. These commonly operate solely based on the interests of the community.

- **For-profit (FP) organizations:** Also known as proprietary, these are investor-owned. Their operation must consider the interests of their investors.

Both types of organizations also differ in their financial-planning capabilities and decision-support analyses. For-profit entities usually have more real-time data accessible for more robust and agile decision making. Non-profits are learning from this model as competition in healthcare becomes more prominent and organizational consolidation continues.

Another way the U.S. healthcare industry differs from other industries is that most revenue comes from payments made to providers of healthcare services (that is, hospitals and medical providers) by third-party payers (that is, commercial insurance companies or governmental programs). In most other industries, payment is made by a customer of a business. In healthcare, "customers" include a vast group: payers, employers, suppliers, and recipients of the services (consumers). This complexity makes it difficult for the primary customer (the patient) to understand and compare the true cost of healthcare services.

Finally, employers play a key role in the purchase of group health insurance offered to employees, which in recent years has shifted to high-deductible plans. These plans shift costs for services from the employer to the employee. These plans have also facilitated the collection of co-pay and co-insurance for services rendered at the time of service versus waiting for payment. These changes have further strained the system for both providers and consumers of U.S. healthcare.

The Affordable Care Act (ACA) of 2010 has reportedly narrowed the gap between those who are medically insured and those who are not. With currently changing U.S. leadership and legislation, it is anyone's guess as to whether this outcome will remain. Will all Americans have health coverage? Will there be a continued need for the challenged governmental payment programs of Medicare and Medicaid? Will prices rise for those who are already insured?

Read more about the ACA at https://www.healthcare.gov/where-can-i-read-the-affordable-care-act/ or http://kff.org/health-reform/fact-sheet/summary-of-the-affordable-care-act/.

Conclusion

Accurate financial records are imperative. Not only do they reflect all current and past business activity, but they provide a useful accounting of accomplishments (and failures) to be considered when planning for the future. Business planning is an iterative process. It never really ends. Unexpected occurrences, unintended consequences, and uncontrollable environmental factors are the norm.

The following is a series of suggested "rules" developed over nearly four decades in healthcare and business. The concepts presented in this chapter coincide with many of these learned examples:

- **Rule 1: Finance is the language of business:** Learn how to use the financial concepts presented in this chapter to build a business case for what you need or want to accomplish in your leadership role.

- **Rule 2: Cash is king:** Cash provides any business (or person) with options. Lenders typically don't lend money to people who can't manage it.

- **Rule 3: Money talks:** If you can make a positive financial impact in your organization, it will provide you with many more opportunities for career growth.

- **Rule 4: Sometimes, you have to spend money to make money.** Invest in people, education, and training. These activities should not merely be viewed as a cost, but as an investment in the future with a predicted solid return of investment.

- **Rule 5: Leadership is important:** Approximately 50% of any company's results can be directly tied to the leadership (Waddill-Goad, 2013). Leaders make positive contributions to organizations by using good judgment and making sound financial decisions.

- **Rule 6: Use Donabedian's structure/process/outcome model:** This model was first applied to quality but also can drive finance. For more on this model, see Chapter 8, "Innovation in Nursing."

- **Rule 7: A thousand small things make a bigger difference than one big thing:** Every small decision that adds impact helps! Treat the company's money like it is yours—don't waste it.

- **Rule 8: Become an operations expert:** If you learn how things really work, you can get things done!

- **Rule 9: More is not always better:** Look at the entire structure and process for efficiency, efficacy, and synergy. Adding more resources can sometimes just make a bad problem worse.

- **Rule 10: Innovation is critical to healthcare success:** Be creative! Many of the old ways of doing things just don't work anymore.

CONCEPT CAPTURE

The following link provides access to a short interview (less than 15 minutes) on YouTube by the Harvard Business Review (HBR) with Joe Knight, author of *Financial Intelligence:* https://www.bing.com/videos/search?q=what+managers+need+to+know+utube+video+&view=detail&mid=3820B890BB80B843F6CB3820B890BB80B843F6CB&FORM=VIRE.

The video discusses what all managers (or leaders) need to know about finance and how Knight teaches people to read financial statements and about finance to develop financial literacy. Note that Knight, co-owner of the Business Literacy Institute, also blogs frequently on the topic of financial literacy at http://www.business-literacy.com/all-about-bli/blog/.

4

COMPETENCY IN BUSINESS

Competency in business encompasses many diverse topics. No one is really ready for all the differing aspects of assuming a leadership role or becoming an intrapreneur or entrepreneur. Experiential learning, along with selected formal educational courses, can often be a winning combination. It is wise to proactively learn about the aspects of business before launching a new business. Attempting to learn along the way can result in a number of unnecessary mistakes.

"Competence, like truth, beauty, and contact lenses, is in the eye of the beholder."
–Laurence J. Peter

Obtaining the Correct Expertise

Whether you're an entrepreneur in a small business or an intrapreneur in a larger organization, one of the most important things is to know your limits of competency. A great deal of expertise in numerous areas is required to legally, efficiently, and successfully run any type of business. Passion goes a long way, but business-related ignorance can produce a plethora of problems. Many intrapreneurs and entrepreneurs aren't sure when and how to get help.

Schreiner (2016) describes *business competency* as a set of skills that allow for success in the world of business. Without these skills, leaders and/or business owners may find their experience more difficult than it needs to be. Schreiner (2016) says some competencies are innate, whereas others can be learned or developed with a concerted effort and provides the following list of five suggested areas of competency for business owners or leaders (Schreiner, 2016):

- **Organizational comprehension:** Understanding the structure and hierarchy within and around the chosen business environment is crucial.

- **Financial understanding:** Because the true nature of business is about making money, financial acumen is vital for sustainability.

- **Management skills:** Communication, relationship skills, and leadership skills are essential for success.

- **Technical competencies:** One example is being proficient in information technology, which is pervasive in today's world.

- **Personal characteristics:** Rejection is common in business. Charisma, self-confidence, and high self-esteem can enhance resilience in the face of this rejection.

All business leaders must know their strengths, identify what they are good at, and focus on what they like to do. Ultimately, all other business-related tasks can be insourced (that is, delegated to someone else in the organization) or outsourced (sent to outside professionals).

- *Insourcing:* Insourcing works best when you build an in-house team of committed experts. When their incentives are aligned, these individuals can share a similar passion and overall vision for work.

Often, large organizations are filled with employees with untapped expertise. For effective teamwork, you must get to know co-workers to identify strengths and potentially gain access to their network of resources.

- *Outsourcing:* Some business ventures may require outsourcing, or collecting a team of external professionals with specific expertise who can be retained for specific situations in which their type of expertise is necessary.

Networking is an especially good way to find outside professionals who complement internal expertise.

Following is a list of professional experts who are often helpful to business leaders:

- Attorneys
- Accountants
- Insurance brokers
- Bookkeepers

- Information technologists

- Marketing, graphic design, and media experts

- Administrative assistants

- Colleagues with differing expertise

- Business, life, and health coaches

- Healthcare providers (to ensure health and well-being)

Regardless of the organizational structure, alignment is critical, whether you seek to achieve a specific small goal or meet challenges relating to the larger organizational mission, vision, and values. Emphasizing this alignment—communicating it to link each member's contribution to the whole—is essential for business success. So, too, is recognizing and rewarding the accomplishments of top team members. This often motivates others to succeed.

One type of entrepreneur is the so-called *solopreneur.* A solopreneur is a "one-man show"—someone who personally carries all the same responsibilities as other small or large businesses. For solopreneurs, it is especially important to connect with others to avoid feeling isolated. This includes joining local, state, and national trade associations; attending professional conferences; engaging in strategic learning opportunities; and volunteering time and talent to build meaningful relationships in business. Since there is no one to delegate to, solo business owners must also think strategically about where best to spend their limited amount of available time. For more information on solopreneurs, see the article "4 Differences Between Solopreneurs and Entrepreneurs Working Alone" by John Rampton at https://www.entrepreneur.com/article/245766.

Core Competencies

In their book *The Value-Added Employee* (2001), Cripe and Mansfield listed 31 core competencies. Although this publication is somewhat dated, these competencies remain relevant for both intrapreneurs and entrepreneurs. They are grouped and listed in Table 4.1.

TABLE 4.1: ESSENTIAL CORE COMPETENCIES

People Competencies	
Leading Others	*Communicating and Influencing*
Establishing focus to communicate relevant information to others	Attention to global communication
	Oral communication
Providing emotional support to enhance others' commitment to their work	Written communication
	Persuasive communication
Fostering teamwork	Interpersonal awareness
Empowering others	Influencing others
Managing change	Building collaborative relationships
Developing others	
Managing performance	Customer orientation

Business Competencies	
Preventing and Solving Problems	*Achieving Results*
Diagnostic information gathering	Initiative
Analytical thinking	Entrepreneurial orientation
Forward thinking	Fostering innovation
Conceptual thinking	Results orientation
Strategic thinking	Thoroughness
Technical expertise	Decisiveness

continues

TABLE 4.1: ESSENTIAL CORE COMPETENCIES (CONTINUED)

Self-Management Competencies
Self-confidence
Stress management
Personal credibility
Flexibility

As the world rapidly changes, work-related roles are without exception fraught with numerous challenges. Processing the onslaught of constant information and ever-changing priorities makes it difficult to focus. Possessing a set of diverse skills, such as the ones listed here, provides an arsenal of tactics for anyone in business.

> *"I have always looked at my competencies before accepting any responsibility."*
> –N.R. Narayana Murthy

Setting Boundaries

Feelings of overwork and exhaustion have become the new normal in the world of work and business. This thinking stems from a long recessionary environment, where workers are now required to do more with less. In recent decades, downsizing, rightsizing, layoffs, forced early retirements, and so on have fueled the mindset among workers that anyone is expendable and can be effectively replaced. It's no wonder workers are driven to keep up—sometimes to an obsessive extreme!

At the same time, Hougaard and Carter (2016) have observed a new phenomenon in the general population, called *action addiction*. They argue that this deep-rooted condition, caused by chemical imbalances in the brain, has resulted in constant busyness. However, this busyness is about chasing short-term wins and derails people from reaching their larger goals. Hougaard and Carter believe this action addiction is in fact a new form of advanced laziness—one in which people are so preoccupied with these "busy" tasks, they avoid being confronted with larger questions such as the following:

- Am I working in the right career?

- Am I present with my children?

- Is my life purposeful?

- Am I climbing to reach the top of a ladder that is leaning on the wrong wall?

As an intra- or entrepreneur, it is easy to be completely consumed by what appear to be necessary business activities to ensure success. Indeed, were it not for the need for sleep, many would work around the clock. Hence, learning to set effective boundaries is important. The bottom line is that many workers trade too much time in their life for too little at their jobs. We cannot manufacture more time, so we must use it wisely.

Many studies in the literature showcase the effects of stress, being overburdened with work, etc. It is well known that tired workers can be dangerous and that productivity is not only affected by long hours worked but by a cumulative effect of this behavior. To combat busyness, we must be willing to place ourselves in a "timeout" by injecting space into our busy lives and pausing our efforts to complete a never-ending to-do list. Busyness and action addiction are choices. We must be sure we are busy doing *the right* things, not just *a lot of* things. And, breaks should be a priority when we need them.

Recently, lawmakers in France have attempted to combat the blurred lines between work and home by enacting legislation to tackle work-related burnout. Essentially, this new law—although not without controversy—gives French workers the "right to disconnect." It is designed to counteract the increase in work-related stress and its association with digital technology as described by Mosbergen (2016). Lawmakers hope this will result in a work culture in which doing more with less is no longer the norm.

Solopreneurs, intrapreneurs, and entrepreneurs must become expert at balancing their myriad responsibilities. They must pace themselves; show technical expertise; be experts at networking, communication, influence, persuasion, environmental awareness, sales, and marketing; form strategic partnerships; be credible; be forward thinkers; and build diverse alliances—all while keeping in mind their own well-being. After all, if you lose your health, all your work will be for naught.

When it comes to setting hard boundaries between their work lives and their personal lives, entrepreneurs and solopreneurs often have a more difficult time than intrapreneurs. These types are almost always thinking about *something* related to business, seem to have an endless supply of ideas and things to do, possess a passion for improvement and innovation, and are interested in complex problem solving. However, these people are generally not addicted to just *doing*; they seek to produce results.

"Put gaps in your life: moments to reflect, prepare, meditate, and breathe."
–Jody Adams

MINDFULNESS IN BUSINESS

In recent years, numerous U.S. companies have taken note of the benefits of *mindfulness,* defined by Kabat-Zinn and quoted by Meister (2015, para. 2) as "paying attention in a particular way; on purpose, in the present moment and non-judgmentally." This practice has been used with success to lower healthcare costs, improve employee productivity, augment employee focus, and reduce work-related stress (Meister, 2015). Indeed, in his book *Mindful Work: How Meditation Is Changing Business from the Inside Out* (2015), Gelles profiles transformative results in companies that adopt mindful practices, including leadership integration for decision-making (that is, ensuring everyone is on the same page when making decisions).

Being mindful takes training and practice. As mentioned, the mind has a propensity to be busy at all times. On top of that, both our society and the advent of digital technology have potentiated the speed with which information becomes available. To combat this, everyone should take time to rest, do nothing, and consider meditation to allow space in the mind for better thinking, creativity, and more thoughtful action. Most decisions are better made through timely intentional thought than reactive action.

Remaining calm, focused, and composed amid a chaotic environment is essential in healthcare and business—and it's a skill set that can be learned. It takes patience to lead others and to think carefully before you speak. The best leaders throughout history exhibited awareness through emotional intelligence, were perceptive, and were tuned in to their own intuition. Examples in the U.S. include the leaders in office during the 9/11 terrorist attack, the Oklahoma bombing, various school shootings, and other major events in history.

Leadership

BusinessDictionary defines *leadership* as "the individuals who are the leaders in an organization, regarded collectively" (Leadership, n.d.). According to that same source, the term *leadership* may also refer to "the activity of leading a group of people or an organization or the ability to do this." A leader is someone who "steps up in times of crisis, and is able to think and act creatively in a variety of difficult situations." In addition, being a leader means doing the following (Leadership, n.d.):

- Establishing a clear vision

- Sharing that vision with others so they will follow willingly

- Providing information, knowledge, and methods to realize that vision

- Coordinating and balancing the conflicting interests of all members and stakeholders

In business and in life, rarely does everything go according to plan. Good business leaders can quickly and confidently adjust when plans go off the rails, identifying their weaknesses (and the weaknesses of others) with precision for course correction. In today's turbulent business world, continual learning and the ability and fortitude to make strategic adjustments on the fly are essential.

Unfortunately, much of what is required of business leaders cannot be taught—qualities like talent, temperament, initiative, intuition, agility, and a willingness to take risk. Still, leadership-development initiatives are important. After all, nobody knows *everything*. And it's always wise to research topics that you don't know much about and/or gather additional perspectives. More often than not, formal education, seminars, conferences, and networking lead to new areas of learning and fresh opportunities for everyone involved.

All too often, development is overlooked both in small business and in larger organizations. Alternatively, organizations leave these types of initiatives to human-resources personnel, in which case they are often not based on relevant data and are viewed as a cost rather than an investment for the future.

WOMEN IN BUSINESS

Women have made tremendous strides in all fields of industry. However, elements of the famous "glass ceiling" remain. Indeed, according to research conducted at three major U.S. universities, being a woman is still perceived as a negative in business, and men are viewed as better entrepreneurs (Shane, 2015). This research also revealed that when people formulate an image of what an entrepreneur looks like in their mind, that entrepreneur is nearly always male. These perceptions potentiate gender inequality and pose challenges for leaders and policy makers at all levels.

Hewitt (2014, p. 132) observes that women in business must walk a fine line. For example, consider the following contrasting qualities:

Too self-aggrandizing	Too self-deprecating
Too aggressive	Not assertive enough
Too opinionated or shrill	Unable to command the room
Too blunt or direct	Too nice
Bloodless	Hysterical
Too provocatively dressed	Too frumpy
Looks too young	Looks too old

According to Hewitt, women who display too many of the qualities listed on the left are often perceived as negative, while women who display too many of the qualities listed on the right are seen as too nice.

Fair or not, to succeed in today's business world, women must be better than their male counterparts. They must be fearless, exude confidence, exhibit grit, and persevere. At the same time, they must be "likable" (Packard, 2016).

This can be a tough row to hoe, but the benefits make it worthwhile. Brooks (2014) notes that new research findings show that teams do in fact benefit from the addition of women in business, especially in the areas of creativity and collaboration. However, this is true only when competition does not does not dominate the mix. According to Brooks, research shows that women generally do not like to engage in conflict—indeed, doing so may actually decrease their creativity— whereas men often prefer going head-to-head in business situations.

*"[T]he best teams I've encountered have
one important thing in common:
Their team structure and processes
cover a full range of distinct
competencies necessary for success."*
–Jesse James Garrett

Creativity and Problem-Solving

Historically, traditional academic programs in all specialties did not
allow for much creativity in the curricula. For example, in nursing, it
focused on learning tools such as case studies and clinical scenarios to
train nurses to problem-solve by looking for deviations in the norm.

With advances in simulation and revised curricula, however, this is beginning to change—and that's a good thing. Gamification (better known
as *gaming*) principles have become an effective translator of knowledge
and application in multiple industries. For example, Deloitte (a provider
of business and financial consulting) developed a gamified program
called *DLA* for its employees using content from top-tier business
schools hosted in a fun online environment. (You can read more about
it here: https://hbr.org/2013/01/how-deloitte-made-learning-a-g.)

In general, healthcare has been slower to adopt technology than many
other industries. However, that is changing. Innovation by those outside
of healthcare striving for better services and systems will change the face
of healthcare as we now know it. Nursing, being both art and science, is
beginning to apply more creativity to problem-solving. Some problems
in healthcare have persisted over decades. However, nurses are now
being empowered to solve a host of problems using innovative thinking
in clinical settings, business settings, product development, care coordination, care delivery, as well as many other areas (Tsai, Liou, Hsiao, &
Cheng, 2013).

In recent years, psychometric scholars have devised tools to measure creativity, including factors that may or may not influence creativity that help to identify its origin: learned or innate. Each of these methods aim to identify linkages with environmental factors and personality traits (Mindgarden, n.d.).

Because of recent and ongoing changes within the healthcare industry, nurses face new problems for which old solutions are neither applicable nor effective. This means that creative thinking in nursing will become even more important. Although nursing care has changed little in the last several decades (except for the use of new technologies), it will likely need to evolve in order to remain sustainable. Based on population and age statistics, futurists predict record numbers of patients will need care in the years to come. A system mired in the past will not be a successful system of the future.

For nurses to be creative in their problem-solving, they must work in a supportive environment—one that seeks innovation. The best problem-solving occurs when nurses collaborate with colleagues to devise unique solutions to common problems.

Conclusion

The topics in this chapter require a certain level of introspection about skills and an assessment of competence in relation to business. Being mindful of gaps and taking action are necessary for improvement and to attain competency. Continual learning and a willingness to learn new things are imperative to success in any leadership role and in business. Awareness of the environment and the ability to accurately assess what and who surrounds you are also key elements to ensure business success.

CONCEPT CAPTURE

Many of the concepts in this chapter require further investigation for the most current, the best, or evidence-based practices. Consider taking an inventory of existing skills to determine an effective approach to building a well-rounded team. The following websites provide helpful resources for competency assessment related to business acumen:

- **Society for Human Resource Management (SHRM): Leadership Competencies:** https://www.shrm.org/Resources AndTools/hr-topics/behavioral-competencies/leadership-and-navigation/Pages/default.aspx

- **SalesDog: Competencies in Business Development:** http://www.salesdog.com/bonus/John_Brennan.pdf

- **University of Victoria: Build Your Skills (includes an overall competency assessment and associated worksheets):** http://www.uvic.ca/coopandcareer/career/build-skills/

- **Chron: List of Core Business Competencies to Run a Business:** http://smallbusiness.chron.com/list-core-competencies-run-business-25222.html

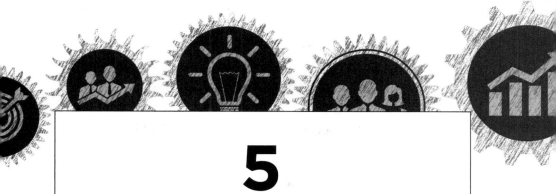

5

MARKETING

Marketing is the process by which goods and services move from a concept to the customer. It involves the coordination of four basic activities (Marketing, n.d.):

- Identifying, selecting, and developing a product
- Determining the price
- Selecting a distribution channel to reach the customer
- Developing and implementing a promotional strategy

One key aspect of marketing is viewing the product or service from the customer's viewpoint. That means asking—and answering—the following questions:

- What do people want?

- What demonstrates value?

- What are people willing to pay for?

This chapter covers some key areas of marketing that are critical for business owners.

"Our job is to connect to people, to interact with them in a way that leaves them better than we found them, more able to get where they'd like to go."
–Seth Godin

Developing a Marketing Strategy

When starting a business, business owners must determine an overarching marketing strategy to make the new business known to the right population of people (that is, the desired market segment). Developing a marketing strategy means answering several key questions:

- What is the business message?

- What services will be offered?

- How will the business be branded? (For more on branding, see the section "Branding" later in this chapter.)

- Will the business be independent or a collaboration? For example, suppose an advanced practice nurse wants to set up her own clinical business. Would she set up the business such that she sees patients collaboratively with a physician? Or would she work solely on her own (within the law and scope of practice, of course)?

- Will the business include consulting? Using the same advanced practice nurse example, would she put herself up for hire to provide specialty services such as infection prevention, business operations, quality improvement, or perhaps risk management?

- What makes the business special or unique in the field of interest?

- Is there competition? If so, how is this business different from the competition?

- Does the business owner have a specific set of skills, a novel concept, or unique qualifications and/or training?

- Is the owner known as an expert in her field? For example, has she received advanced academic preparation or is she nationally certified?

- Will this business serve a niche market?

Market Segmentation

To market effectively, business owners must know who their customers are (or could be). What audience do you want to reach? If you want to establish a business, you must understand the community you want to serve.

One way to do this is through market segmentation, or dividing the total potential customer base into smaller segments. Business owners might use behavioral preferences, geography, demographics (such as age distribution), or psychographics (grouping potential customers relative to attitude, aspirations, etc.) to segment the market and/or for better market research (Market segmentation, n.d.).

Market segmentation is similar to the community assessments nurses perform during their formal nursing education while completing courses related to public health. The same information nurses glean from local health departments—including data points that relate to ethnicity, illness, composition of family units, levels of poverty, cause of death, and existing healthcare providers—can be used in numerous other ways. For example, these public health data can be used to determine the kinds of services needed in a particular area. It could also signal the best location in the community for a certain type of business. And, depending on the location, it could offer insight in establishing a pricing strategy. For example, if you want to open an aesthetic practice, offering Botox and cosmetic fillers, it will likely be unsuccessful in a community that is poverty-stricken. If, however, it is offered in a community with a more affluent population, it could be quite successful.

> *"People don't buy what you do,*
> *they buy why you do it."*
> –Simon Sinek

TWO TYPES OF MARKETING

Kagan et al. (2015) describe two types of marketing:

- **Internal marketing:** With internal marketing, a company markets to its own employees. These employees are seen as both internal customers and marketing agents to promote the business.

- **External marketing:** External marketing means marketing to people outside the business. That is, external marketing involves making the public aware of the products or services offered.

Creating a Marketing Plan

Chapter 2, "Business Infrastructure," noted the importance of a marketing plan. A typical marketing plan outlines two main points:

- How to reach the target market segment (customers)

- How to engage the target market segment to buy or continue to buy your products and/or services

According to Lavinsky (2013b) of Growthink, a formal marketing plan should include the following sections:

- **Executive summary:** This is a comprehensive overview of the sections in the plan.

- **Target customers:** This section of the marketing plan describes the demographic and psychographic profiles of the population you are trying to reach, as well as their predicted needs and wants as they pertain to the products or services you will offer.

- **Unique selling proposition:** This section distinguishes your company from the competition. It could be a tagline that identifies the brand. (For more on branding, see the section "Branding" later in this chapter.)

- **Pricing and positioning strategy:** These strategies must be aligned for optimal performance in the chosen market.

- **Distribution plan:** This section details how customers will buy products or services from you.

- **Offers:** This section includes special deals to drive new customer traffic and/or secure return customers.

- **Marketing materials:** These are collateral used to promote the business, such as a website, digital media, printed materials for distribution, and so on.

- **Promotion strategy:** This section describes how you will advertise the business—for example, via television, billboards, press releases, written material, event marketing, etc.

- **Online marketing strategy:** These days, customers begin their search for products and services by searching online. That means you must develop a strategy to capture those customers. Four key components of an effective online marketing strategy are keywords, search engine optimization (SEO), paid online advertising, and social media. (You will learn more about using social media in your marketing efforts later in this chapter.)

- **Conversion strategy:** This section outlines how you plan to turn prospective customers into paying customers—for example, through sales tactics or social proofing (testimonials).

- **Joint ventures and partnerships:** This section lists intentional relationships built to monetize the business venture.

- **Referral strategy:** A strong customer referral base is one of the best ways to establish a business. It lends credibility and creates a pipeline of growth.

- **Transaction pricing:** It is important to set and monitor pricing using available data sources, such as market value, competition analysis, bundling strategies for pricing efficiency, etc.

- **Retention strategy:** Searching for new customers must be balanced with retaining current or past customers for return purchases. Customer loyalty is crucial.

- **Financial projections:** This section outlines the expected results of your business venture.

> *"The best marketing doesn't feel like marketing."*
> –Tom Fishburne

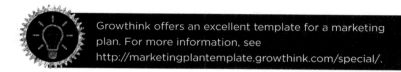

Growthink offers an excellent template for a marketing plan. For more information, see http://marketingplantemplate.growthink.com/special/.

To explore the marketing plan further, let's use the example of the aesthetic practice we mention in the previous section. For this type of business, the targeted market segment includes people who might be persuaded to enhance their appearance via subtle changes using inject-able substances. To reach this target audience, the business might adver-tise at health clubs, boutiques, salons, and other similar businesses. (As an added bonus, building relationships with these types of businesses can facilitate the sharing of customer contacts.) In addition, word-of mouth advertising, or referrals, from existing customers is invaluable. The key to generating this type of advertising is building connections and relationships with others.

Generating Good Marketing Ideas

Remember the show *Bewitched*? It aired during the 1960s and 1970s. The show was about a young witch named Samantha who married a New York ad executive named Darrin. Many episodes showed Darrin sitting in the family's den drawing up ad campaigns. Amazingly, cam-paigns that would have taken Darrin all night to design can now be done almost instantly thanks to digital media. Still, despite these and other changes, the need for good marketing ideas remains.

What is a "good" marketing idea? A good marketing idea is one that effectively gets its message across to the community of people who are most likely to buy your product or service. This community might be as narrow as in your geographical location or networking circle, or as wide as the entire country or even the world.

As you seek to generate marketing ideas for your business, study ads that capture your attention. Ask yourself:

- What do you like about them?

- Are they more formal or casual?

- Are they designed in a classic, humorous, or trendy fashion?

- What draws you to each of them?

- What is it that makes you think about them even when you aren't seeing them?

Chick-fil-A has an incredibly recognizable advertising campaign, using cows to sell chicken. Few people can pass a Chick-fil-A billboard, most of which feature cows who appear to have painted a sign that reads "Eat Mor Chikin" (with its characteristic misspellings), and fail to recognize that Chick-fil-A is actually selling chicken. (It doesn't hurt that their products are delicious!)

Another example of a recognizable marketing campaign is that of the University of Texas MD Anderson Cancer Center, which places a red strike through the word *Cancer*. This conveys a visual message—and an extremely powerful statement—to all who view their brand of products and services (cancer treatment). The message is that cancer can (and, hopefully, will) be eradicated if a patient chooses to be treated at MD Anderson.

Often, the first impression a person receives about a business is through its marketing campaigns. Evidence indicates that first impressions, carved from brief exposures, form lasting impressions (Flora, 2004). For this reason, it's critical to ensure that these first impressions of your business and brand are positive. Like they say, you don't get a second chance to make a first impression!

Identifying Marketing Channels

There are several channels through which you can broadcast your marketing message. Traditional channels include billboards, radio, television, bus stop benches, and even clothing. As mentioned, there are online channels, too, including social media (discussed in the next section).

But that's not all. When it comes to marketing channels, a little creativity goes a long way. For example, consider a recent campaign, called "Deliver Happiness," by online shoe retailer Zappos. In this campaign—which was widely viewed as revolutionary—Zappos partnered with American Airlines and Houston's George Bush International Airport to convert baggage-claim carousels into giant roulette wheel–style game boards. Each carousel was covered with slogans and images of prizes, such as shoes, jackets, backpacks, and home appliances. If a traveler's suitcase landed on an image of a prize, a rep from Zappos would hand that prize to the traveler (Feloni, 2013; MediaPost, 2013). The cost of the campaign was minimal compared to the impact it made on travelers in the airport and the national news exposure the campaign generated.

When it comes to marketing campaigns and advertisements, it's essential to meet people where they are. That's why bail-bond companies place ads outside every jail, local restaurants place ads in literature distributed by hotels to guests, and sunscreen companies advertise at swimsuit shops.

> *"Good marketing makes the company look smart. Great marketing makes the customer feel smart."*
> *–Joe Chernov*

SMARTPHONE ADVERTISING

Anderson (2015) reported that research by the Pew Research Center revealed that 68% of Americans own smartphones—an increase of almost 100% in just 4 years. Indeed, smartphones are quickly becoming all-purpose electronic devices, especially for mobile and tech-savvy 18- to 29-year-olds, as evidenced by a decrease in home-computer ownership in this same population from 88% in 2010 to 78% in 2015 (Anderson, 2015). Not surprisingly, these people are not reading advertisements in the elevator, signs in the lobby, or billboards on the streets, because their eyes are on their phones! This is exactly the type of opportunity savvy marketers look for. People may be looking for restaurants, personal services, or things to do on their phone, and marketers should provide them. Today, this could be done through pop-up advertisements—that is, "push" marketing, where items you have searched for in the past instantly appear when you search for something new or new ads appear after you download the latest apps; through text messages from retailers; through banners that appear on a section of your smartphone screen or in social media feeds; and more.

Easy (and cheap) ways for nurse entrepreneurs to raise their profiles include connecting with local and national organizations, placing themselves on lists of recommended people who possess specific expertise, becoming credentialed in a nursing specialty, and making themselves known in social circles that can influence their businesses.

Marketing via Social Media

Social media connects people. It opens a whole new world. Thanks to social media, people all over the globe can quickly and easily share their lives with others. Millions of Americans use some type of social-media platform to connect, keep up with others, and share their views with the outside world.

Social media platforms like Facebook, Twitter, Instagram, LinkedIn, Snapchat, and YouTube aren't just great sources of social engagement, however. They're also great platforms for marketing and advertising.

Indeed, for business owners and marketers, social media represents nothing less than a marketing revolution.

Using social media in your marketing efforts yields a number of benefits, as described by DeMers (2014b) in his "Top 10 Benefits of Social Media Marketing":

- **Increased brand recognition:** With social media, you can syndicate content and increase brand visibility.

- **Improved brand loyalty:** Recently, Texas Tech reported positive results for companies that engage in social media. Higher customer loyalty may result when companies use social media tools to directly connect with their customer audience.

- **More opportunities to convert:** Every post represents an opportunity to gain a customer or engage with current customers.

- **Higher conversion rates:** Brands become humanized by interaction via social media.

- **Higher brand authority:** Interaction with social media followers can help businesses develop a following.

- **Increased inbound traffic:** Without social media, you or your brand may be limited to those who already know you.

- **Decreased marketing costs:** In its most basic form, social media is essentially free.

- **Better search engine rankings:** Being active on social media can improve your search engine rankings.

- **Richer customer experiences:** Social media is a real-time communication channel that enables customer interaction, which can enrich their experience.

- **Improved customer insight:** Businesses that use social media may gain valuable information about customer preferences and other important insights.

> *"The best way to predict the*
> *future is to create it."*
> *–Peter Drucker*

In addition, search engines can optimize advertisements submitted via social media (to better find you). In addition, these advertisements can generate secondary revenue each time someone views or clicks it. Finally, you can gather and assess data about how much traffic the business's social media profile generates, shown by geographic area, by "friend" status, or from search criteria. Simply put, if used in the right way, social media can propel a business to the next level!

Some nurse entrepreneurs rely on research and formal publications for exposure. But as Shawn Achor, author of *The Happiness Advantage* (2010) humorously notes, academic-published research articles are generally read by only seven people—and one of those is probably your mother! Using social media can help nurse entrepreneurs raise their profile.

Deciding which social media platform will work best for your business may take a bit of time and research. Must-have social media platforms depend on the nature of the business and what type of customer you are trying to reach. To help you investigate your social media options to find the best match for your business, Levy (2013) provides a brief overview of relevant platforms here: https://www.entrepreneur.com/article/230020. In addition, Manafy (2014) describes her perspective on these companies here: http://www.inc.com/michelle-manafy/how-to-choose-the-best-social-media-sites-to-market-your-business.html.

Although there are no real rules for using social media, it is not without risk. Just as social media can make you instantly famous for being an expert or providing a quality product or service, it can also make you instantly infamous for lying or saying something stupid. Anything you post on social media will be almost impossible to permanently delete.

There are no take-backs. Just as you must think before you speak, you must think before you post anything to social media. You must also take care when linking your business or brand with others via social media. Avoid linking with others who are unknown to you (what if they turn out to be a criminal?), have a negative work or personal history, or support something you or your business does not.

COMMENTS

Social media is a two-way street. That is, for anything you post, you may receive comments. These comments can be positive or brutally negative—or anything in between. But that's not all. Even if you *don't* post something on social media, you may find yourself or your business in the cross-hairs of other social media users.

Proctor & Gamble discovered this the hard way. During the late-2000s, it launched a marketing campaign for its Always brand of feminine products. Its slogan: "Have a happy period." This slogan was not well received by some very vocal women (customers). They felt it was wrong to portray a menstrual cycle as "happy," and shared their disgruntlement via social media. As more and more women chimed in, Proctor & Gamble found itself in full crisis-management mode!

Social media, like everything else, must be used with caution.

As with other marketing channels, social media presents lots of room for creativity. For example, in recent years, various businesses have aligned with several YouTube stars, who are extremely popular among teens and tweens (EngagementLabs, 2015). According to *Forbes* (Berg, 2015), one of these stars, who goes by the handle PewDiePie, raked in some $12 million in 2015 in exchange for his ongoing commentary on video games. Some businesses have tapped these YouTube stars to serve as celebrity spokespeople and to feature their products in their videos, giving them entrée to a very desirable market.

"Creativity is intelligence having fun."
–Albert Einstein

Branding

Branding is an important marketing concept. But what is it? In simple terms, "your brand is your promise to your customer" (Williams, n.d., para. 2). It stems from "who you are, who you want to be and who people perceive you to be" (Williams, n.d., para. 2). Maybe you want your business to be seen as innovative. Or experienced. Or luxurious. Or budget-conscious. Whatever description you choose, it informs your brand.

Karen Post, also known as the Branding Diva, likens branding to "brain tattooing." It's the art and science of planting your unique essence in the minds of the buying market (Post, 2015). In simpler terms, it's getting people to remember you and what you sell.

To define your brand, ask yourself these questions (Williams, n.d.):

- What is the mission of your company?

- What features or benefits do your products or services offer?

- What do your current and prospective customers think about your company?

- What qualities do you want your current and prospective customers to associate with your company?

Successful brands are perceived to be honest, to show integrity, to be good at what they do, to be professional, and to deliver quality results.

Williams (n.d.) offers these suggestions for effective branding:

- Design a solid logo and put it anywhere you can.

- Develop messaging that communicates your brand.

- Integrate your brand into every aspect of your business—how you answer your phones, what salespeople wear on sales calls, your office décor, and so on.

- Develop a brand voice that reflects your brand, whether it's friendly, formal, or something else, and use it in every communication.

- Create a memorable tagline—a concise statement that captures the essence of your brand.

- Standardize your marketing materials to reflect your brand and ensure that all these materials share the same look and feel.

- Be true to your brand. Otherwise, your customers won't be true to you.

- Be consistent. There should be no confusion around your brand.

 If you brand your business effectively, you'll find that you draw customers in more easily and may even be able to charge more for your product.

The brand doesn't apply only to the business. It applies to the business owner, too. Business owners should possess a winning leadership "cocktail" of people skills, communication abilities, and influence over others, combined with a reputation for high performance (Leland, 2016). In short, they should demonstrate executive presence—a combination of gravitas, communication skills, and professional appearance, exhibited by confidence, decisiveness, integrity, emotional intelligence, vision, and reputation. And of course, you must dress and act the part. After all, would you trust an infection-prevention nurse with long, false fingernails and chipped nail polish? Would you trust a chef who walked out of the kitchen unshaven, unwashed, with dirt and/or stains on his uniform? Would you trust a physician who smells like cigarettes and alcohol? Would you trust a teacher whose English is packed with slang, poor sentence structure, and bad grammar? Being a clean, polished professional is one of the most important things a business leader can do. Remember: Your image is your brand.

THE IMPORTANCE OF CREDIBILITY

Credibility is an important feature of any brand—and of business in general. Consider the example of the aesthetic practice. To draw customers, that business would likely want to distribute before and after pictures of its clients to prove that it gets results. (Such a business would also benefit from developing a brand that expresses the notions of natural beauty and confidence, as well as attainability.) Similarly, nurses who perform interim leadership services might publish a detailed list of credentials, professional experiences demonstrating results, and reputable references on their website. And legal case review and/or expert witness nurses would likely publicize their client list, as well as other measurable metrics or statistics such as cases won, lost, or settled.

Conclusion

Marketing can be fun! Business owners must think creatively and explore a variety of options to determine the best approach. Be flexible and take risks to see what works, and if your approach *isn't* working, then change course. The important thing is to find what marketing media works best for you and/or your business. Experimentation with differing strategies (and their subsequent results) will point you in the right direction!

CONCEPT CAPTURE

To determine whether your marketing concept is appropriate and effective, reflect on your answers to the following questions:

1. What message do you want to send with your marketing?
   a. Who are you?
   b. What service(s) do you offer?
   c. What makes you the most qualified to offer this service to your clients?
   d. Why are you the best choice?
2. Who is your audience?
   a. What population will use your business services?
   b. Where is that population located inside your community?
   c. What similar services exist in your community?
   d. What complementary services exist in your community?
3. How will you send the right message?
   a. What message best matches your personality and your business?
      i. Humorous
      ii. Pristine and polished
      iii. Elegant
      iv. Casual
   b. Where might your audience best find your message?
      i. Movie theater ads
      ii. Billboards
      iii. Magazines/newspapers
      iv. Radio/television
      v. Social media
   c. What opportunities are there to think outside the box?
      i. Can you sponsor local community events by donating money or volunteering your time and support in exchange for advertising?

    ii.   Can you sponsor local charity fundraising events?

    iii. Can you offer free services for selected community groups (for example, free school physicals for the local high-school football team or cheerleading squad, free legal advice for cancer patients needing help with living wills or power of attorney paperwork, etc.)?

4. How will you know what marketing is most effective?

   a. Should you survey your clients to identify how they learned of your service?

   b. Should you track clicks on social media sites or Internet ads?

5. What is your assessment of market equilibrium/ saturation?

   a. Is there demand beyond the current supply? (If so, there is room for growth.)

   b. Can customers afford the the product or service should they demand it?

   c. Are similar businesses successful and able to survive with competition? (Is there room for you in this market?)

6

LAUNCHING A PRIVATE APN PRACTICE

Since the implementation of the Affordable Care Act (ACA) in 2010, and with an increasingly diverse, aging population and a growing shortage of primary care providers, advanced practice nurses (APNs) have assumed more responsibility for ensuring timely access to high-quality healthcare (Duncan & Sheppard, 2015). Indeed, the professional responsibility of APNs has morphed into clinical autonomy, requiring increased decision-making skills for diagnosis, treatment, and evaluation (Facchiano & Snyder, 2012). Thanks to their educational preparation and the variety of clinical practice settings in which they work, APNs are well positioned to offer new and innovative ways to improve access to healthcare, improve quality of care, and decrease the overall cost of care (Gutchell, Idzik, & Lazear, 2014).

For more information about the ACA—specifically, a timeline that shows how and when provisions of the act will be implemented—visit http://kff.org/interactive/implementation-timeline. Note, however, that this legislation may be overturned and/or significantly changed by a new U.S. Presidential administration in the year 2017.

Given these healthcare industry changes, it is perhaps not surprising that more and more APNs have launched their own private or independent practices. There are boundless opportunities for APNs who want to practice independently. In addition, running an APN specialty practice can be rewarding in many ways. Designing a practice to meet patient needs, providing patient-centered healthcare, and doing it in a way that is creative and innovative can benefit patients, staff, and providers alike.

Private practice also comes with barriers and challenges, however. The complexities of self-employment can be daunting. APNs looking to open a practice must be aware of national standards, as well as the individual state laws governing practice. More than half the states in the U.S. have Nurse Practice Acts that restrict APNs from practicing to the full extent of their knowledge, education, and certification (Duncan & Sheppard, 2015). These limitations vary from state to state and may come in the form of restrictions on prescriptive privileges, on the ability to sign for referrals, on the ability to determine disability status, on the full completion of worker's compensation forms, and on the ordering of home healthcare or durable medical equipment (DME) for patients. In addition, APNs may also be required to have collaborative practice agreements with physicians (Duncan & Sheppard, 2015). Nevertheless, starting a private practice can be an exciting adventure that leads to a fulfilling and rewarding career.

*"I've missed more than 9,000 shots in
my career. I've lost almost 300 games.
Twenty-six times I've been entrusted
to take the game's winning shot
and missed. I've failed over and over
again in my life and that's why I succeed."*
–Michael Jordon

Some state laws impede nurse practitioners (NPs), certified nurse midwives (CNMs), and certified registered nurse
anesthetists (CRNAs) from launching their own expanded
or full practice (Duncan & Sheppard, 2015).

A REAL-WORLD PRACTICE

Dr. Charlotte Mason in Jackson, Wyoming owns a private APN practice
that offers health and wellness services for families, preventive care,
urgent care, commercial driver license (CDL) medical exams, drug and
alcohol testing for local and national companies, veteran evaluation
services, and occupational health screenings. (She is fortunate because
Wyoming offers nurse practitioners an expansive scope of practice,
most likely due to geographic limitations.) Since the clinic's inception,
it has added an aesthetic component and a line of skin care products
to complement the medical services. The practice also rents space to
visiting medical providers.

Other examples of real-world practices include one APN who opened a
truck-stop clinic along the interstate (I-70) to offer CDL health screenings and general medical care to long-haul truckers. Another APN
contracts her services for locum or temporary assignments all over the
world. She has worked in such places as Thailand, the Aleutian Islands,
Antarctica, and the South Pole station.

Credentialing

In July, 2008, the Advance Practice Consensus Work Group and the National Council of State Boards of Nursing (NCSBN) APRN Advisory Committee released a report calling for consensus in the regulation of the roles of APNs. The purpose of this report was to provide continuity of licensure, accreditation, credentialing, and education (LACE) for APNs to improve patient safety, improve mobility of ANPs across state borders, and improve access to care (APRN Joint Dialogue Group, 2008; Rounds, Zych, & Mallary, 2013).

The outcome was the creation of the LACE Consensus Model. This model provides a unified approach to APN credentialing. LACE stands for (American Nurses Association [ANA], 2009):

- **Licensure:** This is the granting of the authority to practice.

- **Accreditation:** This is the formal review and approval by a recognized agency of educational degree or certification programs in nursing or nursing-related programs.

- **Certification:** This is the formal recognition of knowledge, skills, and experience demonstrated by the achievement of standards that are identified by the profession.

- **Education:** This is the formal preparation of APRNs in graduate-degree granting or post-graduate certificate programs.

This model serves to (Elliott & Walden, 2015):

- Decrease ambiguity regarding the APN scope of practice

- Enhance quality of care and access to care

- Provide a systematized, clearly depicted description of APN expectations

The LACE protocol outlines the minimum entry to practice elements for APNs. Additional requirements are set by city and state laws, hospitals, insurance companies, and individual state boards of nursing and pharmacy.

In addition to these, APNs in private practice need an Employee Identification Number (EIN) and Medicare and Medicaid provider numbers. (Because Medicaid is state regulated, APNs must complete separate applications if they intend to file with adjoining states.) They must also complete any credentialing processes with private insurance companies. Some insurance companies require that providers have admitting privileges at area hospitals to be considered preferred providers or designated as in-network, so it is important for providers to become credentialed with hospitals near their practice site (Watson, 2015). Admitting and rounding privileges are individually governed by hospital and medical staff protocols as well as state law.

A hospital affiliation can strengthen the relationship between APNs and hospital-based providers (Watson, 2015).

To perform low-risk office diagnostic testing, such as rapid strep or influenza, urine dip sticks, urine pregnancy, or blood sugar, APNs require a Clinical Laboratory Improvement Amendment (CLIA) waiver certificate. In addition, additional training and certification requirements may apply for the administration of urine drug screening, breath alcohol testing, Nexplanon insertion, or intrauterine device (IUD) insertion. And of course, APNs must comply with city and state licensure requirements to conduct business.

For more information about CLIA certification, see https://www.cms.gov/regulations-and-guidance/legislation/clia/certificate_of_-waiver_laboratory_project.html.

According to Kleinpell, Hravnak, & Hinch (2008), APNs must be prepared to submit the following:

- References

- Work history

- A state-controlled substance registration number

- A Drug Enforcement Administration (DEA) number

- A National Provider Identifier (NPI)

- Proof of licensure

- A National Registry of Certified Medical Examiners number (if planning to perform CDL medical exams)

- Copies of educational degrees

- Certification for basic life support techniques (cardiopulmonary resuscitation/advanced cardia life support/pediatric advanced life support/advanced trauma life support)

- Liability insurance for the entire practice

- Collaborative practice agreement, including details for the collaborative medical doctor (MD) if necessary, per the requirements of each individual state

- Organizational memberships

- Continuing education units (CEU) by year, including details of the type of education received

- Immunization status

- Certification verification

- Any disciplinary action (historical or in effect)

- Any concerns of health or disabilities that may impact care provided

- Practice privileges requests (specific procedures)

- Practice protocols (evidence-based practice [EBP] protocols used)

Growthink offers an excellent template for a marketing plan. For more information, see http://marketingplantemplate.growthink.com/special/.

Keeping track of all these certificates, licenses, and so on can be a somewhat daunting task. Maintaining a master list can be helpful, and keeping a file (physical or computer) for information about continuing education, insurance, licenses, certificates, due dates, and all the rest is a must. In a small or solo office, it may be up to the clinician to maintain these records. For a larger practice, an office manager can be tasked with this job. Additional outside resources, such as an independent human resource services provider, may be useful for their expertise.

In an entrepreneurial nursing business, it is the responsibility of the licensed nurse to ensure he or she abides by legal standards and professional and specialty nursing standards. These are most often found in recent healthcare literature and within each state's scope of practice, determined by the official licensing authority (Koch, 2016).

> *"It's not about ideas.*
> *It's about making ideas happen."*
> *–Scott Belsky*

Fostering Evidence-Based Practice

APNs spearheading independent practice should foster an environment rich in evidence-based practice (EBP). EBP is the integration of the best research evidence resulting from well-designed studies using clinical expertise and patient values (Melnyk, Gallagher-Ford, Long, & Fineout-Overholt, 2014). Before the 1970s, healthcare providers relied very little on EBP in decision-making (Facchiano & Snyder, 2012). Instead, decisions regarding patient care were often based on anecdotal or outdated information or on tradition. "This is the way we have always done it," was a common statement made by those charged with training young doctors and nurses. It wasn't until the 1990s that EBP really took hold.

In 2001, The Institute of Medicine (IOM) issued a statement calling for patient-centered care based on accurate, timely, and up-to-date clinical information that reflected the best available evidence (Olsen, Aisner, & McGinnis, 2007). The statement also encouraged healthcare providers to individualize treatment based on patient needs, resources, and beliefs; to employ quality improvement (QI) strategies; and to use informatics in care and practice (Facchiano & Snyder, 2012).

The IOM envisioned a healthcare system that (Olsen et al., 2007):

- Draws on the best evidence to provide care most appropriate for each patient

- Emphasizes disease prevention and the promotion of health

- Delivers the most value

- Adds to learning throughout the delivery of care

- Leads to improvement in the nation's health

There are EBP protocols available for nearly all health conditions, such as diabetes, heart failure, arrhythmias, chronic obstructive pulmonary disease (COPD), asthma, pneumonia, anticoagulation, and more. However, these are just guidelines. Each unique patient must be evaluated to provide the best, most appropriate care. For instance, when caring for a frail, 87-year-old woman with diabetes, hypertension, and osteoporosis, it might not be appropriate to insist she maintain a hemoglobin A1c of 6.5% (which is the recommended target for persons with diabetes). In this case, the risk of hypoglycemia and the potential for falling far outweighs the long-term effects of elevated blood sugar. Hence, individualized care is required.

As easy and sensible as it sounds to incorporate EBP into everyday patient care, it is still not the standard of care for most real-world practices (Melnyk et al., 2014). Clinicians cite numerous reasons for not using EBP in day-to-day patient care. These include the following (Melnyk et al., 2014):

- Time constraints

- Lack of knowledge and skills

- Lack of resources to access EBP guidelines

- Lack of management support

- Resistance from colleagues

APNs who operate an independent practice must overcome these barriers and ideally implement best-practice strategies into their business model. An excellent way to encourage the use of EPB by team members is to promote interest in, understanding of, and the value of evidence-based, standardized protocols. Additionally, including staff in the formation of practice protocols improves participation.

As the leader of a practice, you can facilitate the process by following several basic steps (Aasekjær, Valen Waehle, Ciliska, Nordtvedt, & Hjälmhult, 2016):

1. Introduce a basic understanding of EBP among providers and staff.

2. Formulate an answerable question in the PICOT format (see the following sidebar).

3. Search for the best evidence available using peer-reviewed, robust research reports.

4. Critically review and evaluate research for validity, reliability, and clinical applicability.

5. Integrate evidence into practice using clinical expertise, individual patient needs, patient values, and circumstances.

6. Evaluate outcomes.

7. Disseminate the protocols into practice.

---

*"There's nothing wrong with staying small.
You can do big things with a small team."*
–Jason Fried

PICOT

- *Patient population of interest:* What patient population or problem are you trying to address?

- *Intervention or issue of interest:* What will you do for the patient or problem?

- **Comparison with another intervention/issue:** What are the alternatives to your chosen intervention?

- **Outcome of interest:** What will be improved for the patient or problem?

- *Time frame:* At what time following the intervention do you decide it is doing more good than harm?

(Thabane et al, 2009)

Practices can employ electronic systems such as UpToDate, Epocrates, and PubMed, which offer access to EBP content. Indeed, many of these systems enable clinicians to import teaching materials into their documentation or progress notes and print them for patient-education purposes. Additionally, evidence-based calculators such as the American Heart Association Cardiovascular Risk Calculator, The Gupta Perioperative Cardiac Risk Calculator, and Calculate by QXMD provide easy access to tools that support evidence-based decision-making (Goff et al., 2013). The use of these and other evidence-based tools arms providers with easy access to evidence-based guidelines, regardless of their location or practice size, and saves time.

 You can read more about cardiac risk calculators from the American Heart Association (AHA) here: http://news.heart. org/aha-acc-reaffirm-new-cardiovascular-prevention-guidelines-risk-calculator/.

Coding, Billing, and Reimbursement

Coding, billing, and reimbursement generally prove challenging for most healthcare providers. This is because it is extremely complex. Entire books have been written on the subject of evaluation and management (E&M) coding alone! Still, all patient visits must be properly accounted for to ensure practice compliance, not to mention business success. Therefore, although it's true that it never hurts to hire an expert billing company, all providers and staff within a practice should be familiar with the intricacies of coding, billing, and reimbursement (Marting, 2015).

Family practice providers survive within a slim margin of profit (Evans et al., 2015). Yet in general, providers tend to unwittingly under-code, resulting in thousands of dollars in lost revenue (King, Sharp, & Lipski, 2001). Proper coding also reduces the number of denied claims, which is critical to any practice. Estimates indicate that at current rates, each claim denial costs approximately $25 to rework. Due to the amount of work involved, as many as half of all denied claims are never refiled (Marting, 2015).

COMMON REASONS FOR DENIED CLAIMS

Insurance claims might be denied for a number of reasons. According to Marting (2005), these may include the following:

- **Missed filing deadlines:** Claims must be filed in a timely manner.

- **Incorrect or outdated patient insurance information:** Be sure the patient's insurance information is up-to-date and the numbers are entered accurately.

- **Improper diagnosis coding:** Documentation in the medical record must support the selected codes. Medical documentation templates can be useful tools for ensuring the use of appropriate codes (Sage, 2014).

- **Failure to capture charges:** Be sure to code for all care provided and know what is legally allowable.

- **Not knowing which services are bundled in a specific type of payment:** Some services are bundled with others.

- **Improper use of modifiers:** Of particular note are modifiers 25 and 59. Modifier 25 refers to a separately identifiable service provided by the same provider, to the same patient, on the same day as another procedure or service, with a global fee period. Modifier 59 pertains to global procedures where the same provider is responsible for both components of the global fee (the professional *and* the technical component).

- **Inconsistencies in data submission:** This might include billing an adult under a pediatric code or attributing a female code to a male patient.

Office staff must be diligent to minimize preventable losses. In addition, APNs should review all denials within their practice setting. These reviews should encompass reason(s) for denial, which insurance companies are denying certain claims, and the percentage of refiling success.

Appropriate coding and accurate billing are not only essential to the financial success of a practice, they are legally mandatory (Evans et al., 2015). A lack of knowledge or understanding about coding and billing regulations is not a defense for failure to comply. Fraud—whether intentional or not—may result in fines, loss of privileges, and/or disciplinary action (Adams, Norman, & Burroughs, 2002). Both up-coding (to enhance income) and under-coding are considered fraud.

Compassionate healthcare providers may be tempted to under-code in an attempt to help self-pay or low-income patients. This is a mistake. Coding is required per the established visit guidelines. However, coding and charging are two very different things. As the owner or leader of a practice, you may choose to discount the *charges for service*.

For prescheduled patients, it's best to gather co-payment information, determine which services the payer will cover (such as wellness exams, mammography, etc.), obtain authorization for services to be rendered, and note any deductible limitations *before* the patient arrives. In addition, to avoid claim denials for incorrect insurance or demographic information, the practice should ensure this information is correct at each patient encounter (Crocker, 2006). Finally, Medicare patients should have an Advanced Beneficiary Notice (ABN) of non-coverage signed prior to undergoing any testing or procedures that might not be covered by Medicare. This notice informs Medicare patients that they may be personally responsible for certain charges not reimbursed by Medicare (Centers for Medicare & Medicaid Services, n.d.). This advance work will streamline the practice's overall workflow and prevent delays when the patient is ready to exit. That being said, sending billing statements between 30 and 45 days after the visit might prompt patients to work with their insurance providers to resolve any benefit issues that may result in out-of-pocket payment from the patient (Aasekjær et al., 2016; Crocker, 2006).

Coding, billing, and reimbursement are incredibly complex. It's a good idea to establish a network of resources for coding support—for example, similar practices or consultants (Crocker, 2006). You should also take advantage of continuing education offerings that address the intricacies of the ever-evolving world of coding and billing. Finally, professional organizations like the American Association of Nurse

Practitioners (AANP) are excellent resources for coding guidance. The link to the AANP's website is https://www.aanp.org/.

Patients often are unaware of the various aspects of their health plan. This includes required co-payments, deductible information, pharmaceutical coverage, exclusions, and so on. Collecting all this information before the patient visit enables the practice to collect any money owed at the time of service (provided the patient has sufficient funds) and avoid filing delays.

> *"If you're not a risk taker, you should get the h*** out of business."*
> –Ray Kroc

Risk Management

For any business owner, greater independence brings greater risk. Developing a risk-management plan—to be followed by all providers and staff—is crucial to protecting the practice. For the ANP-owned practice, risk management is ultimately about minimizing the chances of an adverse outcome, protecting the patient from harm, and providing the best quality of care, thereby shielding the practice from litigation (American Academy of Family Physicians, n.d.).

One obvious form of risk management is insurance. For maximum protection, the practice will likely require multiple types of insurance coverage. One main type is malpractice insurance. Malpractice insurance usually covers the owner(s) of a practice and typically extends beyond the boundaries of the office setting. Note, however, that many malpractice insurance plans that provide coverage for nurses and APNs do not cover physicians or physician assistants who might work within an APN practice, may not cover a practice that employs either of these, and may not cover non-nurse clinicians. Be sure to fully investigate the appropriate insurance(s) for your chosen type of business prior to start-up.

Insurance types, coverage, and rates vary state to state, and can be very costly. With any type of insurance, be sure to verify the expanse of coverage.

Other types of insurance might include commercial, property, automobile, life, health, disability, personal liability, etc., depending on the type of practice or business entity. In addition, depending on the legal structure of the practice—for example, if it is a partnership—you might choose additional insurance to cover you in the event normal business operations are disrupted (for example, your partner dies). Finally, depending on the size of your business, you may also be required to provide insurance benefits to employees in accordance with the ACA. (Offering insurance has the added benefit of helping with employee recruitment and retention.)

To set an appropriate rate, insurers will need to know how many providers, nurses, unlicensed medical providers, and non-medical employees your practice employs.

Another form of risk management is thorough and accurate documentation in the medical record. A comprehensive documentation strategy is your greatest defense against patient misunderstandings and/or potential litigation. Documentation of all patient or client encounters—including phone messages, billing correspondence, appointment reminders, consults (whether formal or informal), referrals, record requests, and refusal of recommendations—can be important evidence in a court of law (CNA, 2010).

It is particularly important to document interactions with patients—especially the provider's thought process in issuing a diagnosis. This information will be necessary should a conflict arise (Achar & Wu, 2012). For example, suppose a patient complains of low back pain following a fall. The provider might conclude through a careful history and physical exam that the cause of the pain is a muscle strain. In that case, an appropriate diagnosis and code would be "strain of muscle, fascia, and tendon of lower back, initial encounter (S39.012A)". Assuming no further diagnostic testing is indicated or performed, it would be essential to document the provider's thought process (Achar & Wu, 2012)—for example, "low suspicion of fracture based on age of patient, mechanism of action, no spinal tenderness on exam, and lack of associated symptoms." It would also be wise to include any EBP source information about the diagnosis. For example, per UpToDate guidelines, diagnostic imaging in the early stages of low back pain is not associated with improved outcomes (Achar & Wu, 2012). It would be helpful to note this in the documentation.

Recent years have seen a movement toward electronic data. Indeed, over the past decade, electronic data have significantly improved and standardized documentation. A 2009 survey by the Nursing Service Organization showed that APNs who used handwritten chart notes were twice as likely to be involved in a lawsuit compared to those using an electronic medical record (CNA, 2010). Using templates can help guide practitioners to obtain all important pieces of history, physical, and key documentation for each patient encounter.

A third form of risk management is to simply foster excellent provider-patient relationships. Indeed, this is one of the best ways for providers to shelter themselves against litigation. Providers and patients must both:

- Understand their limitations

- Establish realistic goals by listening to each other

- Be open-minded and non-judgmental

- Show empathy

Patients must be as much a part of the healthcare team as their providers. Feeling respected empowers patients to take ownership and responsibility for their own healthcare and lowers the risk of dissatisfaction.

A key aspect of fostering good provider-patient relationships is ensuring interactions go smoothly. Keep these tips in mind:

- **Use reflective language:** Repeat direct quotes to accurately describe patient feedback.

- **Read between the lines:** Statements like, "I always need an antibiotic so my cold doesn't turn into pneumonia," or "No one has ever been able to figure out what is wrong with me," can illustrate a patient's level of expectation, cooperation, and credibility (Teichman, 2000).

- **Be thorough:** After completing a review of body systems, ask the patient if she has anything to add or additional concerns. This engages the patient and ensures a level of completeness (Teichman, 2000).

- **Be specific when documenting the physical exam:** Avoid generalized terms and refrain from judgmental descriptions. Instead, describe behavior, appearance, mood, etc. Citing specific examples such as, "patient is tearful" or "patient is unable to remain in one position for longer than a few minutes" is best (Teichman, 2000).

- **Offer no guarantees:** Clinicians should avoid giving any guarantees to the patient. Instead, it is better to quote EBP, statistics, and other verifiable information. For example, regarding birth control, it might be wise to convey that when taken correctly, the birth control pill is 99.9% effective.

- **Discuss treatment decisions:** Treatment decisions always warrant a conversation with the patient, including what was or was not done and why, as well as the risks and benefits of treatment, non-treatment, or medication prescribed (Teichman, 2000). Be sure to document the conversation, and note any educational materials given and discharge instructions.

- **Summarize the visit and clarify next steps:** It is always best to give patients a summary of the visit, a plan of care, instructions regarding what to watch for, when to call for further instructions, when to return to the office, or when it might be necessary to go to the closest emergency department if their symptoms fail to improve or get worse.

One easy way for APNs to avoid risk is to only accept assignments for which they are qualified, both educationally and experientially (Koch, 2016).

RISK-MANAGEMENT RECOMMENDATIONS

The following resources include recommendations for risk management. Although they are somewhat dated, the recommendations remain relevant for today's practice:

- **Nurse Practitioner Claims Study (http://www.hpso.com/ Documents/Risk%20Education/individuals/NursePractitioner-ClaimsStudy.pdf):** This links to two studies conducted by insurance providers profiling practice over a decade.

- **CNA HealthPro Nurse Claims Study (http://www.hpso.com/ Documents/Risk%20Education/individuals/rnclaimstudy.pdf):** This includes information about risk-management education and premium reductions.

- **Risk Management Continuing Education Program (http://www. nso.com/risk-education/individuals/earn-continuing-education-credit):** This links to an educational program aimed at reducing risk.

Patient Satisfaction

A literature review by Newhouse et al. (2011) revealed evidence that APNs produce excellent clinical outcomes with high patient satisfaction. Indeed, the authors indicated that the quality metrics reviewed over an 18-year period proved APNs not only achieved the established quality indicators, but they raised the bar to a higher level.

According to the IOM report *Crossing the Quality Chasm: A New Health System for the 21st Century* (2001), measures of patient satisfaction should include the following (Committee on Quality of Health Care in America, IOM, 2001):

- Providing safe care with positive outcomes

- Providing services based on EBP

- Providing services in a timely and efficient manner

- Using finances, supplies, and energy wisely and without bias

Patient satisfaction does not always equal good care. For example, in some instances, if patients are not given what they think they need, they may be unsatisfied.

Prakash (2010) lists eight reasons why patient satisfaction should be important to your practice:

- Patient satisfaction leads to patient loyalty.

- Patient satisfaction improves patient retention.

- Satisfied patients will be less vulnerable to price wars.

- Satisfied patients ensure consistent profitability.

- Patient satisfaction increases staff morale and reduces staff turnover.

- Patient satisfaction reduces the risk of malpractice suits.

- Patient dissatisfaction may potentiate accreditation or licensing issues secondary to complaints that must be fully investigated.

- Patient satisfaction increases personal and professional satisfaction for practitioners.

Add to this the fact that satisfied patients are more likely to refer your practice to others. Remember, however, that word of mouth can be both a wonderful marketing tool and a terrible one. A single happy customer will generate four referrals on average. However, one negative experience is generally communicated to 10 other people (Prakash, 2010). Considering that the loss of one customer due to dissatisfaction can result in a loss of up to $200,000 over the life of a practice (Prakash, 2010), those numbers can quickly add up.

One of the best ways to measure patient satisfaction is to subject them to a post-visit survey. In a practice setting, this survey could be provided as a handout at the end of the visit, via email, or via text message. Or, it could be conducted by telephone. Obviously, as technology advances, so too will the healthcare provider's ability to gain instant feedback. This type of patient communication is critical for understanding care requirements and patient satisfaction.

It is important to initiate a regular review or audit of practice-related data, including documentation, billing, patient satisfaction, patient complaints, and meaningful use (which refers to the use of certified electronic health record technology). There are many electronic tools currently on the market, and staff must be educated and engaged to use outcome data to drive quality improvement initiatives.

MAKING A GOOD FIRST IMPRESSION

First impressions are critical for patient retention. Ensuring office staff are courteous and empathetic when interacting with patients, both over the phone and in person, is crucial. Providing a script or checklist may help ensure consistency and completeness between various staff members when interacting with and scheduling patients (Crocker, 2006).

Your practice should provide new patients with relevant information about the office (such as policies or procedures) and the provider. This information should also include payment and collection policies, including instances when a patient will be responsible for all charges (regardless of insurance coverage). Some providers even go so far as to issue a welcome letter to new patients. This document explains the provider's philosophy of care, office hours, charges for missed appointments, provider availability, medication refill policy (for example, requiring 48-hour notice for prescription refill requests), patient responsibilities regarding co-payment of fees and/or collection procedures, accepted insurance plans, payment arrangements for non-covered services or self-pay patients, interest charged on past due accounts, and how to access care after hours (Crocker, 2006). These documents should be reviewed by a legal professional for accuracy and enforceability prior to use.

Conclusion

Owning and managing an APN practice brings with it numerous rewards and challenges. This chapter only scratches the surface of what is required to be successful. Indeed, for each question answered in this chapter, another one inevitably appears. Examples include:

- What is the best location for a practice?

- Should you rent or own office space?

- Should the practice be solo or multi-practitioner?

- Will insurance be accepted? If so, what types?

- Should you opt in or out of Medicare and Medicaid programs?

- Should the staff be multi-disciplinary (a combination of registered nurses and/or unlicensed personnel) and/or multilingual?

This chapter is by no means a complete list of what may be needed to run a practice. However, staying current with EBP, credentialing, coding/billing issues, risk management, and patient satisfaction will provide a solid foundation for a well-built practice.

CONCEPT CAPTURE

The following questions and suggestions have been devised to stimulate thought about the complexities of owning and operating an APN practice:

- Research is important to assess similar businesses in the geographic area. What might make your practice stand apart from the competition?

- Consult with other APNs who have taken the leap into business. Is there anything they would have done differently if they had the chance to do it over again?

- Think carefully about investing with a partner. Would it be better to be solo? Many say you should select a business partner as thoughtfully as you would select a spouse!

- It is essential to select the appropriate legal structure, documents, and expertise for startup. Do you know your options?

- Assess your expertise in all the areas of business competency in this chapter.

- Generate accurate and thorough documentation.

- Understand the rules of coding and billing.

- Explain, discuss, and ask patients to reflect on what they have learned from patient education.

- Understand that patient satisfaction is not always equivalent to quality care delivery and patient healing.

- Met expectations are set expectations. Be sure to clearly communicate with patients.

7

ADVANCE PRACTICE NURSING IN A NON-CLINICAL ROLE

What is an advanced practice nurse (APN)? Most definitions focus on the clinical role of an APN. However, Terhaar, Taylor, & Sylvia (2016) describe various non-clinical roles for APNs, including administrator, policy maker, informaticist, analyst, and more.

In addition, many APNs occupy leadership roles. These nurses typically possess a managerial title, such as manager, director, executive director, chief, or vice president of a service line, a division, an academic program, or a specified workforce (such as all nurses or clinicians). Leadership, like clinical care, is both art and science (Pipe & Bortz, 2009). Preparation for these leadership roles may include formal education, formal or informal training, on-the-job experiences, mentoring, and so on.

These APNs are well-positioned to work both as intrapreneurs leading existing healthcare organizations, and as entrepreneurs who may start new healthcare ventures or choose to work in health-related consulting.

OBTAINING CERTIFICATION FOR NON-CLINICAL APN ROLES

For non-clinical APN specialties, including the roles cited in this chapter, a separate license is typically not required. However, employers may prefer (or even require) APNs to obtain certification or advanced education to demonstrate subject mastery and/or practice competency. Certification is defined as "a process by which an agency or association grants recognition to an individual who has met certain predetermined qualifications specified by that agency or association" (The Center for Health Services Education & Research, 2009, para. 2). The following certification bodies offer certification exams for APNs at several levels to demonstrate knowledge of precise subject matter in a standardized set of managerial and leadership competencies:

- **The American Nurses Credentialing Center (AACN):** http://www.nursecredentialing.org/certification.aspx

- **The American Organization of Nurse Executives (AONE):** http://www.aone.org/initiatives/certification.shtml

Although the exam content for these certifying bodies differs slightly, either one is generally acceptable in practice.

In addition, numerous graduate programs offer formal education as master and doctoral-level degrees in a variety of specialty areas. These programs offer another excellent way to gain—and demonstrate—the knowledge necessary to take on an APN non-clinical role.

Finally, the Academy for Academic Leadership (AAL) is the preeminent consultancy for individual and organizational leadership development in academic health professions (Academy for Academic Leadership, n.d.). Its mission is to cultivate leadership, foster life-long learning, and improve organizational effectiveness through customized professional development and consulting services and products, mostly for academic institutions. You can read more about it here: http://www.aalgroup.org/.

"If you just work on stuff that you like and you're passionate about, you don't have to have a master plan with how things will play out."
—Mark Zuckerberg

On Leadership

While there is no single definition of leadership, the term often refers to an individual or individuals who are responsible for leading an organization (Leadership, n.d.).

The majority of non-clinical APN roles possess a leadership title and/or responsibilities. For example, Delgado and Mitchell (2016) explored what leadership qualities are important in nursing academia. They began with a review of the literature, but found little published information. Thus, they conducted a scientific survey. Their top findings for desirable qualities for leaders in nursing academia were as follows:

- Integrity
- Good communication skills
- Good problem-solving skills
- Vision
- Fairness
- Motivational ability

Additionally, survey respondents viewed good leaders as having certain innate characteristics, such as intelligence. Thus, in addition to having rigorous academic credentials, professors must now possess leadership qualities to ultimately be successful in teaching students.

The same qualities noted by Delgado and Mitchell (2016) as effective for leaders in nursing academia hold true for leaders in virtually all healthcare organizations.

Leadership is a specialty unto its own. Not everyone can do it, is prepared for it, or succeed at it. Moreover, some leadership skills are innate, whereas others can be learned. Historically, advance practice nursing has pertained mostly to clinicians. The overall concept of advance practice nursing is evolving, however, and has now begun to include leadership roles. This is especially true with the newer doctoral programs for a practice-focused doctorate (DNP) versus a research-focused doctorate (PhD).

In addition to the changes in academia, there are also changes in practice, including the emergence of new types of leadership. One of these is aesthetic leadership. According to Mannix, Wilkes, and Daly (2015), aesthetic leaders positively influence the work environment, resulting in a calm clinical workplace. At its core, strong leadership in a healthcare environment—whether one calls it aesthetic leadership or something else—focuses on healing and nurturing, as well as fostering a healing culture (Pipe & Bortz, 2009).

Given the focus of strong leaders in a healthcare environment, one might view leadership as the global range of behaviors displayed by someone that have an enduring and positive influence on those whose lives are affected by him or her (Pipe & Bortz, 2009).

Both intrapreneurs and entrepreneurs are needed for healthcare system improvement. Changing the future will require a change in thinking. With our "inside" knowledge, we nurses are uniquely positioned to lead transformative change. Can we do it from the inside out? Absolutely. Will it require strong leadership? Yes. Be willing to take a chance and become part of the change!

FOSTERING A POSITIVE CULTURE IN HEALTHCARE

Organizational culture has a tremendous effect on the well-being of caregivers (Brennan, 2017)—and leaders potentiate culture. Links between stress, burnout, and a lack of resilience in healthcare workers and productivity have been recognized for decades. Brennan (2017) suggests organizations be more concerned with workplace demands, stress levels, control of stress, relationships, roles, and the pace of change. Current and future healthcare leaders must be aware of the intricacies of the environment and its impact on workers, and be willing to lead by example to promote health among caregivers.

In addition to affecting organizational culture, leadership can have an effect on patient outcomes, which equates to cost (Wong, 2015). According to Wong (2015), research highlights a clear connection between supportive leadership and positive patient safety outcomes. Indeed, studies conducted primarily over the last 2 decades reveal that leaders with a participative and transformational leadership style, who are trusted by employees (where they feel supported by management), play a significant part in the following patient outcomes (2015):

- Reduced medication errors (according to four out of five studies)

- Decreased restraint use and hospital-acquired infections

- Lower patient mortality (according to three out of six studies)

- Increased staff retention

- Enhanced clinical expertise of staff

- Higher patient- and staff-satisfaction scores

- Decreased length of patient stays

- Improved safety culture and safety behaviors of staff

However, patient-fall and pressure-ulcer data showed mixed results. Still, these outcomes suggest that leadership and the work environment that leaders create (that is, the culture) matter.

Cost pressures in healthcare are abundant and most likely will remain. Therefore, mistakes made in a "learning" or supportive environment are much better than in a punitive environment. No environment is error-free, and patient safety must be a priority. While mistakes can be costly, how leaders handle adversity is telling.

Virtually all healthcare organizations must find ways to be safer, more efficient, and more effective; to eliminate waste; and to avoid wasting customers' time. System reform starts with good leadership.

 The impact of leadership on both nurses and patients is undeniable. Thus, leadership should be a higher priority in organizational planning, execution, and succession.

> *"Don't be afraid to give up the good and go for the great."*
> *–John D. Rockefeller*

Exploring Consulting

Franks (2014) describes nurse consultants as instrumental in any sphere. They use their clinical expertise to lead practice, facilitate change, and monitor effectiveness. Indeed, within organizations, consultants contribute to service delivery, public health policy, policy development, and other areas—all while mirroring expected leadership competencies and improved health outcomes (Franks, 2014). The National Nurses in Business Association (NNBA) agrees, noting that it is nurse consultants who usually identify problems and develop solutions (NNBA, n.d.).

Some of the most common types of nursing consultants are those with expertise in the following:

- Nursing practice
- Operations

- Compliance

- Survey readiness

- Infection control

- Leadership

- Interim assignments

- Training

- Education

- Legal issues

- Customer service

- Pharmaceuticals

- Medical devices

- Technology

- Documentation

- Case management

- Project management

There are numerous consulting firms available to help healthcare organizations. Those who are interested in entering this exciting arena will want to consider the following:

- **Setting rates:** To determine an appropriate rate structure, it is always best to research various sources. One excellent source is Salary.com (http://www.salary.com). Here, you can find salary information for practically any type of job, including nurse consulting work, which can help you set your rates. When you determine a target range, it's wise to check with potential clients to ensure you're both on the same page with regard to compensation. Even though most people are uncomfortable talking about money, it's imperative that you do so. Pricing is always a difficult topic to discuss, but in time, you'll become more comfortable with it, and even learn to negotiate as needed.

It may be the case that your rate will be set by the organizations with whom you work, with what they are willing to pay typically being based upon their own data and/or market research. Many healthcare organizations and academic institutions conduct annual market research to assist in designing objective and competitive compensation programs for employees.

- **Obtaining customers:** Networking is a key strategy for spreading the word about your consulting services. (Be sure to keep an address book of contacts, whether paper or electronic.) Referrals are another excellent method. Finally, in recent years, it has become imperative to develop a presence online and in social media to connect with technologically savvy customers.

- **Developing a brand:** A brand defines a specific company, product, or mark (McLaughlin, 2011). Until your services take hold in the marketplace, your brand will almost certainly be associated with you and what you represent. Chapter 5 discusses the importance of branding in more detail.

- **Negotiating contractual agreements:** A contract clearly outlines the terms and conditions of the work to be performed, creating a foundation from which you and your clients or customers can agree. Having a standard contract template that has been approved by legal counsel is crucial.

The Department of Health and Human Services (HHS) mandates the use of the Business Associate Agreement (BAA) for most contractors in all related health entities. The BAA is a standard contractual agreement that requires covered entities to comply with the rules and regulations regarding protected health information for optimal privacy and security (thus, anyone working for them who may have access to patient information must sign one). For more information about the BAA, see https://www.hhs. gov/hipaa/for-professionals/covered-entities/fast-facts/ index.html. For an example of a BAA, see https://www.hhs. gov/hipaa/for-professionals/covered-entities/sample-business-associate-agreement-provisions/index.html.

- **Selling your services:** According to Tobak (2013), everyone is in sales. He therefore recommends sales training to learn how to connect with others, how to negotiate, and how to close the deal. He suggests the following:

  - Do your homework to understand your customer and what you can offer them.

  - Ask good questions, such as, "How can I help you?", "What are your objectives and goals?", and "Are there any concerns we should address?" And carefully listen to the customer's replies. This is necessary both to build your relationship and to obtain a clear scope of work.

  - Make a genuine connection. Much of business is based on relationships, *period*.

  - Be on the same side. Convince your customers that you can and will make them successful. Then do it.

For some, selling comes naturally. Others must work at it. Fortunately, there are many courses and books on learning how to sell.

- **Assessing client or customer value:** Consultants are paid to get results. (That's why I think they should be called *resultants*.) If you get results for your clients, they'll see you as valuable—and tell others about you.

- **Setting limits and boundaries:** Especially when you first start consulting, setting boundaries is hard. In fact, you could find yourself on call 24 hours a day. Your clients are your bosses, and they may need you at any hour of the day or night (especially across time zones). To the extent that it's possible, try to plan ahead. One approach is to plan even as far as one year in advance, noting in your calendar important events, personal time for recovery, holidays, days of work, and so on. That way, you may be able to avoid being run ragged.

- **Reinventing yourself:** *Reinvention* is defined as "the action or process through which something is changed so much that it appears to be entirely new" (Reinvention, 2017). As the healthcare environment changes, you may need to change with it by reinventing yourself. Alternatively, you might reintegrate rather than reinvent yourself. Reintegrators use their knowledge, creativity, and life experience to change their future path rather than liberating themselves completely from their past (Freedman, 2014). The bottom line? If you are not happy doing what you are doing today, change it.

- **Staying relevant:** Good consultants keep abreast of the latest developments in their industry. One way to do this is to obtain additional formal education. In addition to expanding your breadth of knowledge and building your credibility, this approach allows for fresh professional experiences, new insights, and the opportunity to build meaningful relationships. Less formal education in the form of conferences, short courses, etc. is also effective, offering the opportunity to network, be with like-minded people, and learn new things.

- **Taking care of yourself:** Taking good care of yourself will improve the care you give to others. Ask yourself, what do you need to do your best work? It's a good question—particularly for nurses, who typically don't take the time to consider what they need and instead consider only what everyone else needs from them!

- **Promoting mental health and wellness:** Nursing is a physical, mental, emotional, and spiritual journey. That means it's just as important to take care of your mind as it is to take care of your body. There is a plethora of information in the current literature about mindset, mindfulness, meditation, yoga, etc. to promote health, wellness, and well-being. Consider becoming a student focused on your own well-being.

- **Recharging:** Everyone needs time to rest, recover, and re-energize. That way, you free your mind to generate good ideas! (Think of all the times you've hit on a great idea when you weren't trying to—like in the shower.) To help with this, Pipe and Bortz (2009, p. 36) suggest you self-reflect by asking yourself these questions:

  - How do I feel cared for?

  - How do I express my care for others?

  - What causes me to feel nurtured?

  - How do I replenish myself?

  - How does self-replenishment relate to the leadership service of others?

  - What makes me happy?

  - What are my rituals for letting go of work/obligations at the end of the day?

- Am I growing?

- Am I helping others to grow professionally?

- What brought me to nursing/healthcare?

- What brings me strength?

- What/who inspires me?

- Where do I find joy and meaning?

- What legacy do I hope to leave with my leadership influence?

- What rituals can I build into my daily routine that will help me remember my connection with self and source (such as gratitude)?

"Success seems to be connected with action. Successful people keep moving. They make mistakes, but they don't quit."
–Conrad Hilton

Non-Clinical APNs and Business: A Personal Story

Healthcare needs good leaders both those who have innate talent and those who have been schooled in the world of business. And yet, when I chose a graduate program for business (MBA) over one in nursing (MN or MSN) just over 20 years ago, great controversy ensued. (At the time, it was a novel concept; the norm was to continue learning more in and about nursing, while a brave few chose healthcare administration.) When I made my choice, the dean of a regional nursing program paid me a visit just to ask me why. I told her that I thought if I wanted (or was already in) a job that was responsible for the most employees and the biggest budget in the entire hospital, I'd better learn everything I could about running a business!

Little did I know when I entered business school how much it would affect all areas of my life. The concepts have infiltrated my thinking both in business and in personal decision-making. While I yearned to learn how other businesses worked and how they compared to healthcare, I had no idea how the diversity in thinking would offer new opportunities both in and outside of healthcare. I also had no idea at the time that I would be emancipated from a senior healthcare leadership role and self-employed within 3 years of finishing my business education.

Fast-forward to 2017, and I am about to start my 15th year in business. Having both a clinical and a business degree has been invaluable. Would I have been able to start and sustain a company without learning about business? Most likely not. Have I made mistakes? Yes. Did I recover? Yes. Could they have been much worse? I think so. In the end, I believe I am much more helpful to my clients because of my business education and experience, and I think they would agree. My way of thinking is different. Sometimes I ask difficult questions, and the answers can be incredibly insightful.

I do think business school taught me to think in different ways. Incidentally, it also made much of my doctoral program (in executive leadership) easier, as I was already familiar with many of the concepts and had put them into practice.

Conclusion

Although this chapter does not include everything necessary to be a successful entrepreneur, intrapreneur, or solopreneur in a non-clinical APN specialty, it provides enough information for exploration. Building a successful business enterprise requires proper preparation, credentials, good leadership skills, self-care, the critical evaluation of ideas, and fortitude. The journey may be rocky at times, but there will be a never-ending series of opportunities to learn from along the way.

Awareness and observation skills are key, for both the internal and external environment. The world is changing at a rapid pace, and in business, we must change with it. Avoiding mistakes and learning from your mistakes are equally important. Taking time to reflect on what is and isn't working is essential; and, reinvention may be necessary. Lastly, remember to think about what you need to do your best work!

HELPFUL RESOURCES

For further research into non-clinical roles for APNs, see the following:

- **Salary.com:** http://www.salary.com
- **Nursing License Map—Advanced Practice Nurses:** https://nursinglicensemap.com/advanced-practice-nursing/
- **American Association of Legal Nurse Consultants:** http://www.aalnc.org/
- **National Nurses in Business Association:** https://nnbanow.com/nurse-consultant-faq/
- **The Campaign for Nursing's Future—Nurse Entrepreneurs:** https://www.discovernursing.com/specialty/nurse-entrepreneur
- **Nurse Entrepreneur Network:** http://www.nurse-entrepreneur-network.com/
- **Alan Weiss Consulting Group for Solopreneurs:** https://www.alanweiss.com/
- **Synnovatia:** http://www.synnovatia.com/

CONCEPT CAPTURE

The following are some questions to consider when exploring a non-traditional APN role:

- Are you able to work independently?
- Are you comfortable working alone?
- Are you a risk taker?
- Do you have demonstrated leadership skills?
- Can you sell a product or service?
- Do you have a fear of the unknown?
- Are you stress-tolerant?
- Does the idea of not having a regular job scare you?
- Do you have a good support system?
- Are you motivated to serve others?
- Are you good at solving problems?
- Can you make and execute an effective plan?
- Are you well-connected in your professional environment?
- Do you have skills to offer a service or a product others need or want?
- Do you have enough resources to take the risk of becoming an entrepreneur?

8

INNOVATION IN NURSING

A few years ago, after 2 decades working as a nursing leader in multiple healthcare settings, I noticed something: I, and nearly every other leader I encountered, was frequently fatigued. This led me to hypothesize that nursing leadership roles and fatigue might be related. To test my hypothesis, I designed and developed a national survey about what I term *Leadership Fatigue™*. In the summer of 2013, I distributed this survey to nurse leaders, educators, and consultants across the U.S.

The response rate was overwhelming. I received 595 completed surveys (525 of which were used in my statistical analysis). The results from my study proved my hypothesis to be correct. People in nursing leadership roles were negatively affected by their work, experiencing stress leading to mental, physical, emotional, and spiritual sequelae.

These findings about fatigue among nursing leaders were so striking, I began to speak of them around the country. Not surprisingly, many audience members asked a similar question: "What do we do about this?" This led to yet another project: the publication in 2016 of *Nurse Burnout: Overcoming Stress in Nursing* with Sigma Theta Tau International (STTI). This book, written in a positive tone, focused on strategies to not just cope but to thrive in the chaos-filled work environments that characterize today's healthcare industry.

> *"Innovation distinguishes between a leader and a follower."*
> *–Steve Jobs*

What does this have to do with innovation? I tell this story to serve as an example of innovation. Merriam-Webster (n.d.) defines *innovation* as "the introduction of something new" or "a new idea, method, or device." According to Ness (2015), it's the engine of scientific progress. Innovation is fundamental to change and central to progress. Organizations need innovation to fuel new ideas for fresh products and services. It's a popular topic—so popular, in fact, that a recent Google search yielded some 571 million hits.

Nurses, too, can and should innovate. Indeed, nursing innovation is sorely needed. For some time, members of the healthcare community—and of the public it serves—have widely agreed that transforming healthcare is a top priority in the U.S. (De Groot, 2009). It's true that in many cases, what used to work in healthcare no longer applies. Thanks to their intimate knowledge of systems, patient care, and patient needs, nurses have a unique opportunity to drive healthcare change.

To learn more about innovation, visit https://www.ideo.org. This is the website for IDEO, an award-winning design and development consulting firm. IDEO is committed to solving many of the world's most pressing problems, including those affecting healthcare.

Change Agility

Ness (2015) posits that our habitual ways of thinking are filtered through something linguists call *frames*. She describes a frame as a structure of expectations and assumptions used to interpret new information, which allow us to think and speak in a common set of models. Frames could also be described as patterns of thinking or a set of norms from which people view and interpret happenings in the world around them. Both innovation and creativity require frame-breaking to spur new approaches, novel thinking, and progress (Ness, 2015).

> Not everyone has the same frames. Certain "lenses," such as formal education, different types of skill-based training, various professions enlisting bias, gender, geographic location, and so on, change thinking. And of course, some people's "lenses" are just different because of their make-up. As a result, some people are more prone to be creative thinkers than others.

Humans also have a tendency toward what Gestalt psychologist Karl Dunker called *functional fixedness* (Ness, 2015). This is certainly true in healthcare. Ness (2015) explains that when we are taught to use a particular object a certain way or for a certain purpose, we don't see other ways to use it. This is the antithesis of "out of the box" thinking.

Innovators are different. They are adept at *change agility*. That is, they are not stuck doing things in the same old way. They are critically aware, excel in observation, and think differently (Ness, 2015). They don't fear failure or experimentation. Experimentation provides new insight for differing ways to doing things.

Innovators are often able to apply the practices they observe in one industry to another. For example, in recent years, innovators observed that certain practices in the hotel and entertainment venue industries—such as those relating to customer service, environmental design, work methodologies, and even food selection—could apply to the healthcare industry. This has driven a bevy of improvement initiatives in hospital environments and operations by a number of reputable companies and individuals not necessarily known for their work in healthcare, including Planetree, Fred Lee, Disney, Ritz Carlton, Marriott, etc. Here's more information about efforts by each of these companies:

- **Planetree:** http://planetree.org/

- **Fred Lee:** http://www.patientloyalty.com/

- **Disney:** http://www.prnewswire.com/news-releases/disney-institute-announces-new-healthcare-service-program-as-hospitals-prepare-for-public-reporting-of-patient-scores-124846284.html and https://disneyinstitute.com/blog/tag/healthcare-training/

- **Ritz Carlton:** http://ritzcarltonleadershipcenter.com/consulting/culture-transformation-for-healthcare/

- **Marriott:** http://www.prnewswire.com/news-releases/sodexho-marriotts-at-your-request----room-service-dining-makes-hospital-stays-more-appetizing-75380637.html and http://www.hospitalitynet.org/news/4000772.html

When I studied Lean and Six Sigma at The Ohio State University's Fisher College of Business, I read a book called *Learning to See* by Mike Rother and John Shook. (The book profiles value stream mapping and depicts how a process works, highlighting where it can be improved by adding value and reducing waste.) It then occurred to me that "seeing" is what innovators do. They just see things that others cannot. To learn more about this book, visit https://www.lean.org/BookStore/ProductDetails.cfm?SelectedProductId=9&ProductCategoryId=1&utm_source=google&utm_medium=ad&utm_campaign=ADWORDSGRANTLTS&gclid=CI7h3OGM3tICFUm2wAodcnIK4A.

> *"Without change there is no innovation,*
> *creativity, or incentive for improvement.*
> *Those who initiate change will have*
> *a better opportunity to manage the*
> *change that is inevitable."*
> *–William Pollard*

Change does not come naturally for most people. All change can be hard—whether good or bad. Change is often unsettling, can create underlying anxiety, and can result in unintended consequences. Change theorist Kurt Lewin described a three-stage model that reflects how most people deal with change. The stages of the model are as follows (Nursing Theory, n.d.):

1. **Freezing:** This is the state in which the majority of people reside, most of the time. In this state, no change is afoot. People in this state are comfortable.

2. **Unfreezing:** This is what happens when any type of change must occur. This might be a forced change or a voluntary one. For example, consider what happens when someone loses her job. Suddenly, she must rethink her path and change her mindset about what she viewed as her "normal." During the unfreezing phase, she processes what has transpired and the steps she now needs to take.

3. **Refreezing:** With the passage of time, as people adjust to their new "normal," the refreezing process takes hold.

Large-scale change in nursing and healthcare requires extensive unfreezing. After all, this type of change by definition nullifies many traditions, past practices, and standard ways of doing things, resulting in new, drastically altered, or even completely transformed methods.

How one thinks and views the world is often key to whether change is a positive or negative experience. Indeed, this has become an area of study, called *mindset science*. Neuroscientists in this field study how people think about a variety of topics, and how their thinking affects their lives. Innovators are particularly adept at changing their mindset. These people view each day at work as a sort of "learning lab."

For more information about mindset science, see http://www.mindsetonline.com or do a literature search for current journal articles and recently published books.

System Improvements

One area in healthcare that is ripe for change is systems. System improvements—for example, through the leveraging of technology—can do much to help provide better, more affordable care for individuals and the community at large (Thomas, Seifert, & Joyner, 2016).

While there is much more work to be done, the last decade or so has bought significant improvement in this area. One program, called Transforming Care at the Bedside (TCAB), was particularly notable. This national initiative was spurred by the Robert Wood Johnson Foundation and the Institute for Healthcare Improvement (IHI, n.d.-a). The program, which began in the early 2000s and spanned about five years, focused on these four areas:

- Safe and reliable care
- Vitality and teamwork
- Patient-centered care
- Value-added care processes

This project resulted in many sustainable improvements for participating hospitals, including (IHI, n.d.-b):

- Improvement in rapid response teams (for emergencies)

- Improvement in communication systems, such as the implementation of the Situation, Background, Assessment, Recommendation (SBAR) model

- The introduction of professional support programs

- The introduction of nutritional programs that give patients more autonomy

- The redesign of workspaces and workflows using methodologies from other successful industries (which themselves use the teachings of Lean and Six Sigma).

In addition to TCAB, the IHI has launched other critical campaigns aimed at overhauling healthcare. These include campaigns that pertain to the following (IHI, n.d.-b):

- **The triple aim:** Improving the patient experience of care, improving the health of populations, and reducing the per-capita cost of healthcare

- **Leadership initiatives:** For professional development

- **Patient- and family-centered care initiatives:** Planetree, Medical Homes, and others

- **New outpatient care models:** Spanning the continuum of care

- **Cost and quality initiatives:** Decreasing cost while improving quality

- **Access to healthcare:** Especially for those who are financially challenged

- **Strategic partnerships:** Within and outside of healthcare

- **Centers of excellence:** Designated entities with expertise in certain areas

- **Decreasing hospital readmissions:** Penalties now apply from some payers

---

*"Business has only two functions—
marketing and innovation."*
–Milan Kundera

The work facilitated by the IHI over the last decade is nothing short of amazing. The advances made in patient care and in nursing are astounding. There is no doubt that patients have benefited from these changes!

Another type of system improvement that has made a significant impact in patient care and safety is the development of smart pumps (Blakeney, Carleton, McCarthy, & Coakley, 2009). These pumps save lives by making information available to caregivers at the time and point of service, creating a near-foolproof way to prevent intravenous (IV) drug-dose errors, drug-rate errors, and wrong-drug errors. The team that developed these pumps were true innovators. Many other recent system-improvement innovations have likewise made their mark—the use of mobile technologies, the rise of retail clinics, the provision of concierge medicine, and more.

Each of these innovative improvements represents a *disruptive innovation*—requiring the industry to rethink some aspect of its work—and each resulted in transformational change for the better. Still, many view disruptive innovation as controversial because it disrupts the status quo.

Don't just change for change's sake. Changes should stem from existing standards and practices. The American Nurses Association (ANA) publishes *Nursing: Scope and Standards of Practice,* which describes the who, what, where, when, why, and how of nursing practice. (You can purchase this book here: http://nursesbooks.org/Main-Menu/Standards/Nursing-Scope-and-Standards-3rd-Ed.) This publication can be a helpful starting point for nurses who seek to innovate.

This helps to explain why supporting and sustaining innovation is a significant challenge in a healthcare environment (Blakeney et al., 2009). Other barriers include the following:

- **Complexity of systems:** Many say that the largest problem with healthcare is that it is not really a "system." Rather, it is a complicated network of individual entities loosely tied together to form a whole. Rouse (2008) asserts that the success of traditional systems depends on the ability to decompose and recompose the parts. However, in healthcare, no single person or entity has the power to do so.

- **Trial and error:** Many innovations are developed through trial and error—something that many situations in healthcare do not allow for due to patient-safety reasons.

In recent years, Galloway (2009) described the development of training techniques such as simulation that have now made it possible for nurses to develop skills *without* endangering patients (or themselves). Long a tool for risk management and error mitigation in high-risk industries such as aviation, nuclear power production, and in the military, the use of simulation in healthcare continues to grow.

- **Slow decision-making:** Hierarchical organizational structures rarely make speedy decisions. This has the potential to create a host of problems and frequently inhibits innovation.

These barriers necessitate the need for a supportive environment. For true transformation and sustainable change to occur, the culture of the healthcare organization must foster the process of innovation (Blakeney et al., 2009). Real innovation in healthcare will require both engaged clinicians and leaders who can influence change. Change must be led by committed and enthusiastic individuals who embrace innovation, seek to drive positive change, exude a passion for improvement, and exhibit grit and tenacity.

DONABEDIAN'S STRUCTURE/PROCESS/OUTCOME MODEL

One method used to ascertain healthcare quality relative to structure/process/outcomes is Donabedian's original model (Donabedian, 1988, p. 1745). This methodology can also be aptly applied to business in the same format, where structure is the type of business and associated work, process is how the business will operate based on policy and procedure, and outcomes are usually somewhat predictable based on the structure and process. Recently, Moore, Lavoie, Bourgeois, and Lapointe (2015) profiled Donabedian's healthcare model, observing that improvements in the structure of care should lead to improvements in clinical processes, which should in turn lead to improved patient outcomes. Donabedian's model can be applied in myriad ways, such as a healthcare business structure that drives work processes that result in a particular type of work culture and subsequent business outcomes (either satisfactory or unsatisfactory).

"There is no innovation and creativity without failure. Period."
—Brene Brown

Using Talent to Create a Healthy Work Environment

Innovators are usually quite talented people, and in some cases brilliant. Talent is important. Indeed, according to The Center for Talent Innovation, "full utilization of the global talent pool is at the heart of competitive success" (Center for Talent Innovation, 2017). That's why this organization seeks to "drive ground-breaking research that leverages talent across the divides of gender, generation, geography and culture" (Center for Talent Innovation, 2017).

Nurses—a community of united people who span the divides of gender, generation, geography, and culture—have long been known to use their talent for good, and the public they serve knows it. They have been rated first in an annual survey of the most trusted health professions by Gallup every year since 1999 except 2001, when firefighters topped the list (Advisory Board, 2015). This trust represents an enormous opportunity for nurses to take the healthcare helm to make a positive and lasting difference.

NursingLink (n.d.) lists the top 10 qualities of a great nurse as:

- Communication skills

- Emotional stability

- Empathy

- Flexibility

- Attention to detail

- Interpersonal skills

- Physical endurance

- Problem-solving skills

- Quick response time

- Respect

This list offers unique insight into how nurses might think differently about the design and work processes in future healthy workplaces. Nurses must now take more ownership of their work environments and be permitted to use creative thinking and innovative skills to drive positive change. For this to happen, nursing leaders and other healthcare leaders must be willing to allow experimentation, model flexible thinking, and convey confidence in the workforce.

The American Nurses Association (ANA, 2016) offers resources to provide nurses with strategies to create a healthy work environment. You can find more here: http://www.nursingworld.org/MainMenuCategories/ WorkplaceSafety/Healthy-Work-Environment.

Nurses are also in an excellent position to shift today's mindset of an "ill culture" to a "wellness-focused culture" by serving as role models. Healthy Nurse, Healthy Nation, a new initiative by the ANA, is challenging all nurses (estimated to be 3.6 million in the U.S.) to model good health by becoming a healthy nurse. The ANA defines a healthy nurse as "one who actively focuses on creating and maintaining a balance and synergy of physical, intellectual, emotional, social, spiritual, personal and professional wellbeing" (ANA, 2016, para. 1). In addition, "a healthy nurse lives life to the fullest capacity, across the wellness/illness continuum, as they become stronger role models, advocates, and educators, personally, for their families, their communities and work environments, and ultimately for their patients" (ANA, 2016, para. 1). For more on this initiative, see http://www.nursingworld.org/ MainMenuCategories/WorkplaceSafety/Healthy-Nurse.

Nurses can also use their talents for good in other roles, outside the work setting. For example, they can serve on boards, become members or even officers of professional organizations, donate time to charities or religious organizations, offer pro bono services in the community where they live, and so on. All these offer opportunities to pay it forward to make the world a better place.

> *"Innovation comes from the producer—*
> *not the customer."*
> *−W. Edwards Deming*

Conclusion

Systemic change to promote innovation in healthcare must begin with how nurses are educated and with the environments in which they practice. Change is nearly constant, and we must learn to adapt. In today's world, creative thinkers can influence the healthcare system of the future by fostering stellar work environments filled with talented colleagues and a population focused on wellness.

The aim of this book was to give readers a solid foundation in business as it relates to healthcare. Still, there is much more to be learned with changing laws, standards, regulatory insight, quality initiatives, and more. Innovation in nursing and healthcare will be crucial to sustain progress.

There is no shortage of ways to better the healthcare system. The U.S. healthcare sector is plagued with sky-high costs, unequal access, and erratic quality, and is a major drag on the U.S. economy (Herzlinger, Ramaswamy, & Schulman, 2014). This presents enormous opportunity for entrepreneurial thinking and innovation, especially from those who work closest to the customer (patients) in the healthcare sector.

ONLINE RESOURCES ON INNOVATION

- **The Innovation Learning Network:** http://www.iln.org/

- **The Center for Innovations in Care Delivery at Massachusetts General Hospital:** http://www.mghpcs.org/Innovation/index.asp

- **Consortia for Improving Medicine with Innovation and Technology:** http://www.cimit.org/web/cimit/home

- **Healthcare Innovation Awards:** https://innovation.cms.gov/initiatives/Health-Care-Innovation-Awards/

- **ASU College of Nursing and Health Innovation: Healthcare Innovation (MHI):** https://nursingandhealth.asu.edu/degree-programs/graduate/healthcare-innovation-mhi

- **MakerNurse:** http://makernurse.com/

- **MakerHealth:** http://www.makerhealth.co/

- **Innovating in Healthcare:** https://www.edx.org/course/innovating-health-care-harvardx-bus5-1

CONCEPT CAPTURE

Look around you for examples of innovation. Here are some great ways to start:

- What new ideas have been implemented at your place of employment? Did they stick? Were they revised and reimplemented?

- Think about your creative ideas. Could any of them be implemented and tested in your personal life or at work?

- Look for innovation in your surroundings. This works especially well when you are waiting for something. (I know, it means you have to stop looking at your phone and take a digital recess.)

- Research current innovations in healthcare or your nursing specialty online.

- Use a search engine to search for *innovation* and learn more about it.

- If you travel, innovation examples are abundant. Think of all the examples of innovation in aviation and in auto-rental, hotel, and travel companies to name a few. Could any of them be applied to healthcare?

- Think about problems you would like to solve, such as any nuisances or pet peeves.

REFERENCES

Aasekjær, K., Valen Waehle, H., Ciliska, D., Nordtvedt, M. W., & Hjälmhult, E. (2016). Management involvement—A decisive condition when implementing evidence-based practice. *Worldviews on Evidence-Based Nursing, 13*(1), 32–41.

Academy for Academic Leadership (AAL). (n.d.). *About AAL*. Retrieved from http://aalgroup.org/aal_about.cfm

Achar, S., & Wu, W. (2012, July–August). How to reduce your malpractice risk. *Family Practice Management, 19*(4), 21–26.

Achor, S. (2010). *The happiness advantage: The seven principles of positive psychology that fuel success and performance at work*. New York, NY: Broadway Books.

Adams, D. L., Norman, H., & Burroughs, V. J. (2002). Addressing medical coding and billing part II: A strategy for achieving compliance: A risk management approach for reducing coding and billing errors. *Journal of the National Medical Association, 94*(6), 430–447.

American Academy of Family Physicians. (n.d.). *Risk management and medical liability*. Retrieved from http://www.aafp.org/dam/AAFP/documents/medical_education_residency/program_directors/Reprint281_Risk.pdf

American Association of Colleges of Nursing (AACN). (2011). *Nursing fact sheet*. Retrieved from http://www.aacn.nche.edu/media-relations/fact-sheets/nursing-fact-sheet

American Hospital Association (AHA). (2016a). *Financial fact sheet, payment cuts to hospitals since 2010.* Retrieved from http://www.aha.org/content/16/acahospitalcuts.pdf

American Hospital Association (AHA). (2016b). *Underpayment by Medicare and Medicaid fact sheet.* Retrieved from http://www.aha.org/content/16/medicaremedicaidunderpmt.pdf

American Hospital Association Health Forum, LLC. (2016). *Fast facts on US hospitals.* Retrieved from http://www.aha.org/research/rc/stat-studies/fast-facts2016.shtml

American Nurses Association (ANA). (2009). *Consensus model for APRN regulation: Licensure, accreditation, certification, and education.* Retrieved from http://www.nursingworld.org/cmissuebrief

Anderson, M. (2015, October 29). Technology device ownership: 2015. *Pew Research Center Internet, Science & Tech.* Retrieved from http://www.pewinternet.org/2015/10/29/technology-device-ownership-2015/

APRN Joint Dialogue Group. (2008). *Consensus model for APRN regulation: Licensure, accreditation, certification and education.* Retrieved from https://www.ncsbn.org/736.htm

Berg, M. (2015, November 2). The world's highest-paid YouTube stars. *Forbes.* Retrieved from http://www.forbes.com/sites/maddieberg/2015/10/14/the-worlds-highest-paid-youtube-stars-2015/#5602491f542c

Berry, T. (2013). 10 important quotes about business strategy. *U.S. Small Business Administration.* Retrieved from https://www.sba.gov/blogs/10-important-quotes-about-business-strategy

Bowser, J. (2010, July 20). 8 traits of successful entrepreneurs–Do you have what it takes? *Minority Business Development Agency.* Retrieved from http://www.mbda.gov/blogger/starting-business/8-traits-successful-entrepreneurs-do-you-have-what-it-takes

BrainyQuote. (n.d.). *Financial quotes.* Retrieved from https://www.brainyquote.com/quotes/keywords/financial.html

Branding. (n.d.). *Entrepreneur* online. Retrieved from https://www.entrepreneur.com/topic/branding

Brennan, E. J. (2017). Towards resilience and wellbeing in nurses. *British Journal of Nursing, 26*(1), 43–47.

Brooks, C. (2014, August 14). Want creativity? Don't make it a competition, ladies. *Business News Daily.* Retrieved from http://www.businessnewsdaily.com/6971-women-teams-creative-benefits.html

Business. (n.d.). In *BusinessDictionary.* Retrieved from http://www.businessdictionary.com/definition/business.html

Carlson, K. (2015, February 13). Business education for nurses? *Multibriefs.* Retrieved from http://exclusive.multibriefs.com/content/business-education-for-nurses/medical-allied-healthcare

The Center for Health Services Education & Research. (2009). *What is certification?* Retrieved from http://www.healthserviceseducation.com/WhatIsCertificaton.html

Centers for Medicare & Medicaid Services. (n.d.). *Advance beneficiary notice of non-coverage.* Retrieved from https://www.medicare.gov/claims-and-appeals/medicare-rights/abn/advance-notice-of-noncoverage.html

CNA. (2010). *Understanding nurse practitioner liability.* Retrieved from https://international.aanp.org/Content/docs/UnderstandingNursePractitionerLiability.pdf

Committee on Quality of Health Care in America, Institute of Medicine (IOM). (2001). *Crossing the quality chasm: A new health system for the 21st century.* Washington, DC: National Academies Press.

Cripe, E. J., & Mansfield, S. (2001). *The value-added employee: 31 competencies to make yourself irresistible to any company.* New York, NY: Routledge.

Crocker, J. (2006, October). How to improve your revenue cycle processes in a clinic or physician practice. *AHIMA.* Retrieved from http://library.ahima.org/doc?oid=73917#.WBLXsvkrI2w

Delgado, C., & Mitchell, M. M. (2016, January–February). A survey of current valued academic leadership qualities in nursing. *Nursing Education Perspectives, 37*(1), 10–15.

DeMers, J. (2014a, November 3). 51 quotes to inspire success in your life and business. *Inc.* Retrieved from http://www.inc.com/jayson-demers/51-quotes-to-inspire-success-in-your-life-and-business.html

DeMers, J. (2014b, August 11). The top 10 benefits of social media marketing. *Forbes.* Retrieved from http://www.forbes.com/sites/jaysondemers/2014/08/11/the-top-10-benefits-of-social-media-marketing/#2281d8052a4d

Duncan, C. G., & Sheppard, K. G. (2015). Barriers to nurse practitioner Full Practice Authority (FPA): State of the science. *International Journal of Nursing Student Scholarship, 2.*

The Economist. (2010, March 5). *Are health insurers making huge profits?* Retrieved from http://www.economist.com/blogs/democracyinamerica/2010/03/insurance_costs_and_health-care_reform

Ellevate. (2013, May 28). The secret to putting together an insanely successful team. *Forbes.* Retrieved from http://www.forbes.com/sites/85broads/2013/05/28/the-secret-to-putting-together-an-insanely-successful-team/#2ef0c0a31d5c

Elliott, E. C., & Walden, M. (2015). Development of the transformational advanced professional practice model. *Journal of the American Association of Nurse Practitioners, 27*(9), 479–487. doi:10.1002/2327-6924.12171

EngagementLabs. (2015, November 26). *The YouTube vlogger: Social media's latest career choice.* Retrieved from https://www.engagementlabs.com/the-youtube-vlogger-social-medias-latest-career-choice/

Entrepreneur. (n.d.). *Merriam-Webster online dictionary.* Retrieved from http://www.merriam-webster.com/dictionary/entrepreneur

Evans, D. V., Cawse-Lucas, J., Ruiz, D. R., Allcut, E. A., Andrilla, C. H. A., & Norris, T. (2015). Family medicine resident billing and lost revenue: A regional cross-sectional study. *Family Medicine, 47*(3), 175–181.

Experian Information Solutions, Inc. (n.d.). *Credit score basics.* Retrieved from http://www.experian.com/blogs/ask-experian/credit-education/score-basics/

Experian Information Solutions, Inc. (2015, April 23). *What are the different credit scoring ranges?* Retrieved from http://www.experian.com/blogs/ask-experian/infographic-what-are-the-different-scoring-ranges/

Facchiano, L., & Snyder, C. H. (2012). Evidence-based practice for the busy nurse practitioner: Part one: Relevance to clinical practice and clinical inquiry process. *Journal of the American Academy of Nurse Practitioners, 24*(10), 579–586.

Fair Isaac Corporation. (n.d.). *What is a FICO score?* Retrieved from http://www.myfico.com/credit-education/credit-report-credit-score-articles/

Feloni, R. (2013, November 27). Zappos has figured out how to make waiting for your baggage at the airport fun. *Business Insider*. Retrieved from http://www.businessinsider.com/zappos-travel-happy-baggage-game-2013-11

Financial statement. (n.d.). In *BusinessDictionary*. Retrieved from http://www.businessdictionary.com/definition/financial-statement.html

Flora, C. (2004, May 1). The once-over. *Psychology Today*. Retrieved from https://www.psychologytoday.com/articles/200405/the-once-over

Franks, H. (2014). The contribution of nurse consultants in England to the public health leadership agenda. *Journal of Clinical Nursing, 23*(23–24), 3434–3448.

Freedman, M. (2014, January 1). The dangerous myth of reinvention. *Harvard Business Review*. Retrieved from https://hbr.org/2014/01/the-dangerous-myth-of-reinvention

Fry, R. (2015a, April 25). Millennials overtake Baby Boomers as America's largest generation. *Pew Research Center*. Retrieved from http://www.pewresearch.org/fact-tank/2016/04/25/millennials-overtake-baby-boomers/

Fry, R. (2015b, May 11). Millennials surpass GenXers as the largest generation in the U.S. labor force. *Pew Research Center*. Retrieved from http://www.pewresearch.org/fact-tank/2015/05/11/millennials-surpass-gen-xers-as-the-largest-generation-in-u-s-labor-force/

Fuchs, V. R. (2013, July 11). The gross domestic product and health care spending. *The New England Journal of Medicine, 369*, 107–109. Retrieved from http://www.nejm.org/doi/full/10.1056/NEJMp1305298

Furgison, L. (2016). How to create a unique value proposition. *Bplans*. Retrieved from http://articles.bplans.com/create-value-proposition/

Gallup. (2016, December 19). *Americans rate healthcare providers high on honesty, ethics*. Retrieved from http://www.gallup.com/poll/200057/americans-rate-healthcare-providers-high-honesty-ethics.aspx

Gelles, D. (2015). *Mindful work: How meditation is changing business from the inside out*. New York, NY: Houghton Mifflin Harcourt Publishing Company.

Goff, D. C., Lloyd-Jones, D. M., Bennett, G., Coady, S., D'Agostino, R. B., Gibbons, R., … Wilson, P. W. F. (2013). 2013 ACC/AHA guideline on the assessment of cardiovascular risk. *Professional Heart Daily*. Retrieved from http://circ.ahajournals.org/content/early/2013/11/11/01.cir.0000437741.48606.98

Gutchell, V., Idzik, S., & Lazear, J. (2014). An evidence-based path to removing APRN practice barriers. *The Journal for Nurse Practitioners, 10*(4), 255–261.

Hewitt, S. (2014). *Executive presence: The missing link between merit and success*. New York, NY: HarperCollins Publishers.

Hougaard, R., & Carter, J. (2016, January 12). Are you addicted to doing? *Mindful*. Retrieved from http://www.mindful.org/are-you-addicted-to-doing/

Inc. (n.d.). *Cash flow statement: A breakdown of the cash flow statement, and methods for simplifying the procedure*. Retrieved from http://www.inc.com/encyclopedia/cashflowstatement.html

Internal Revenue Service (IRS). (2016). *Employer ID numbers*. Retrieved from https://www.irs.gov/businesses/small-businesses-self-employed/employer-id-numbers-eins

Intrapreneur. (n.d.). *Dictionary.com*. Retrieved from http://www.dictionary.com/browse/intrapreneur

Kagan, I., Biran, E., Telem, L., Steinovitz, N., Alboer, D., Ovadia, K. L., & Melnikov, S. (2015). Promotion or marketing of the nursing profession by nurses. *International Nursing Review, 62*(3), 368–376.

Kahan, S. (2013, August 7). 3 ways to create value that lasts. *Fast Company.* Retrieved from http://www.fastcompany.com/3015225/leadership-now/3-ways-to-create-value-that-lasts

Kaiser Family Foundation. (2016). *State health facts: Population distribution by age.* Retrieved from http://kff.org/other/state-indicator/distribution-by-age/

King, M. S., Sharp, L., & Lipski, M. S. (2001, May–June). Accuracy of CPT evaluation and management coding by family physicians. *Journal of the American Board of Family Practice, 14*(3), 184–192.

Kleinpell, R. M., Hravnak, M., & Hinch, B. (2008). Developing an advanced practice nursing credentialing model for acute care facilities. *Nursing Administration Quarterly, 32*(4), 279–287.

Koch, G. (2016). The RN entrepreneur who owns their own business. *Oregon State Board of Nursing Sentinel, 35*(3), p.10–11.

Kutscher, B. (2014, June 21). Fewer hospitals have positive margins as they face financial squeeze. *Modern Healthcare.* Retrieved from http://www.modernhealthcare.com/article/20140621/MAGAZINE/306219968/

Lavinsky, D. (2013a, September 6). Executive dashboards: Why every business needs one. *Forbes.* Retrieved from https://www.forbes.com/sites/davelavinsky/2013/09/06/executive-dashboards-what-they-are-why-every-business-needs-one/#384f810d37d1

Lavinsky, D. (2013b, September 30). Marketing plan template: Exactly what to include. *Forbes.* Retrieved from http://www.forbes.com/sites/davelavinsky/2013/09/30/marketing-plan-template-exactly-what-to-include/#8dad48f3b82f

Lavinsky, D. (2013c, October 18). Strategic plan template: What to include in yours. *Forbes.* Retrieved from http://www.forbes.com/sites/davelavinsky/2013/10/18/strategic-plan-template-what-to-include/#478d448b47e1

Lazzaroni, D. (2014, June 19). 75 quotes to inspire marketing greatness. *LinkedIn Marketing Solutions Blog.* Retrieved from https://business.linkedin.com/marketing-solutions/blog/7/75-quotes-to-inspire-marketing-greatness

Leadership. (n.d.). In *BusinessDictionary.* Retrieved from http://www.businessdictionary.com/definition/leadership.html

Leland, K. T. (2016, September 16). How to strengthen your personal and executive presence. *Entrepreneur.* Retrieved from https://www.entrepreneur.com/article/278159

Levy, S. (2013, December 2). How to choose the best social media platform for your business. *Entrepreneur.* Retrieved from https://www.entrepreneur.com/article/230020

Llopis, G. (2011, August 22). 4 skills that give women a sustainable advantage over men. *Forbes.* Retrieved from http://www.forbes.com/sites/glennllopis/2011/08/22/4-skills-that-give-women-a-sustainable-advantage-over-men/#285cf162c973

Manafy, M. (2014, July 9). How to choose the best social media site for your business. *Inc.* Retrieved from https://www.inc.com/michelle-manafy/how-to-choose-the-best-social-media-sites-to-market-your-business.html

Mannix, J., Wilkes, L., & Daly, J. (2015, September). Grace under fire: Aesthetic leadership in clinical nursing. *Journal of Clinical Nursing, 24*(17–18), 2649–2658.

Marketing. (n.d.). In *BusinessDictionary*. Retrieved from http://www.businessdictionary. com/definition/marketing.html

Market segmentation. (n.d.). In *BusinessDictionary*. Retrieved from http://www. businessdictionary.com/definition/market-segmentation.html

Marting, R. (2015, March–April). The cure for claims denials. *Family Practice Management, 22*(2), 7–10.

McLaughlin, J. (2011, December 21). What is a brand, anyway? *Forbes*. Retrieved from http://www.forbes.com/sites/jerrymclaughlin/2011/12/21/what-is-a-brand-anyway/#6a436ec22aa4

MediaPost. (2013, December 2). *When everyone zigs, ZAP!* Retrieved from http://www. mediapost.com/publications/article/214622/when-everyone-zigs-zap.html?utm_ source=feedburner&utm_medium=feed&utm_campaign=Feed%3A+media-creativity+ (MediaPost+%7C+Creative+Media+Blog)

Meister, J. (2015, April 27). Future of work: Mindfulness as a leadership practice. *Forbes*. Retrieved from http://www.forbes.com/sites/jeannemeister/2015/04/27/future-of-work-mindfulness-as-a-leadership-practice/#63d6dd62a41b

Melnyk, B. M., Gallagher-Ford, L., Long, L. E., & Fineout-Overholt, E. (2014). The establishment of evidence-based practice competencies for practicing registered nurses and advanced practice nurses in real-world clinical settings: Proficiencies to improve healthcare quality, reliability, patient outcomes, and costs. *Worldviews on Evidence-Based Nursing, 11*(1), 5–15.

Mindgarden. (n.d.). *Creativity*. Retrieved from http://www.mindgarden.com/35-creativity

Mosbergen, D. (2016, May 25). French legislation suggests employees deserve the right to disconnect. *Huffington Post*. Retrieved from http://www.huffingtonpost.com/entry/ work-emails-france-labor-law_us_57455130e4b03ede4413515a

National Nurses in Business Association (NNBA). (n.d.). *Nurse consultant*. Retrieved from https://nnbanow.com/nurse-consultant-faq/

Newhouse, R. P., Stanik-Hutt, J., White, K. M., Johantgen, M., Bass, E. B., Zangaro, G., ... Weiner, J. P. (2011). Advanced practice nurse outcomes 1998–2008: A systematic review. *Nursing Economics, 29*(5), 1–22. Retrieved from https://www. nursingeconomics.net/ce/2013/article3001021.pdf

Newtek. (2012, January 19). 13 types of insurance a small business owner should have. *Forbes*. Retrieved from http://www.forbes.com/sites/thesba/2012/01/19/13-types-of-insurance-a-small-business-owner-should-have/#3a96f6fd94fd

Office of Inspector General (OIG). (2000, March 16). Publication of the OIG Compliance Program Guidelines for Nursing Facilities. *Federal Register, 65*(52), 14289–14306. Retrieved from https://oig.hhs.gov/authorities/docs/cpgnf.pdf

Olsen, L. A., Aisner, D., & McGinnis, J. M., editors. (2007). Institute of medicine roundtable on evidence-based medicine: Charter and vision statement. From *The Learning Healthcare System: Workshop Summary*. Washington, DC: National Academies Press.

Packard, S. (2015). *New rules of the game: 10 strategies for women in the workplace.* New York, NY: Prentice Hall Press.

Packard, S. (2016). *New rules of the game: 10 strategies for women in the workplace.* New York, NY: Prentice Hall Press.

Perlis, M. (2016, June 6). Forbes survey reveals what millennials really want. *Forbes*. Retrieved from http://www.forbes.com/sites/mikeperlis/2016/06/06/forbes-survey-reveals-what-millennials-really-want/2/#53ab378e5608

Pipe, T. B., & Bortz, J. (2009). Mindful leadership as healing practice: Nurturing self to serve others. *International Journal for Human Caring, 13*(2), 34–38.

Post, K. (2015). *Brain tattoo you: Personal brand assessment.* Retrieved from http://brandingdiva.com/product/brain-tattoo-you-personal-brand-assessment/

Prakash, B. (2010, September–December). Patient satisfaction. *Journal of Cutaneous and Aesthetic Surgery, 3*(3), 151–155. doi:10.4103/0974-2077.74491

Rampton, J. (2014, December 1). 50 inspirational entrepreneurial quotes. *Entrepreneur.* Retrieved from https://www.entrepreneur.com/article/240047

Reinvention. (2017). *Bing.* Retrieved from https://www.bing.com/search?q=reinvention&qs=n&form=QBRE&sp=-1&pq=reinvention&sc=8-11&sk=&cvid=7BA548289D814 2F7A4391E4367BFA0F5

Rishel, C. J. (2014). Financial savvy: The value of business acumen in oncology nursing. *Oncology Nursing Forum, 41*(3), 324–326.

Rounds, L. R., Zych, J. J., & Mallary, L. L. (2013). The consensus model for regulation of APRNs: Implications for nurse practitioners. *Journal of the American Academy of Nurse Practitioners, 25*(4), 180–185. doi:10.1111/j.1745-7599.2013.00812.x

Sage, M. J. (2014). Strategies for coding, billing + getting paid appropriately, 2014 supplement. *The California Academy of Family Physicians.* Retrieved from http://www.familydocs.org/f/14.CodingBillingICD10Supplement.pdf

Schreiner, E. (2016). Examples of business competency. *Chron.* Retrieved from http://smallbusiness.chron.com/examples-business-competency-14019.html

SCORE Association. (2016). *Frequently asked questions about SCORE.* Retrieved from https://www.score.org/frequently-asked-questions-about-score

Shane, S. (2015, June 2). Are men better entrepreneurs? That's the perception. *Entrepreneur.* Retrieved from https://www.entrepreneur.com/article/246815

Start-up [Def. 2]. (n.d.-a). In *The American Heritage Dictionary of the English Language Online.* Retrieved from https://ahdictionary.com/word/search.html?q=start+up

Start-up [Def. 1 & 2]. (n.d.-b). In *Merriam-Webster Online.* Retrieved from https://www.merriam-webster.com/dictionary/start-up

Teichman, P. G. (2000, March). Documentation tips for reducing malpractice risk. *Family Practice Management, 7*(3), 29–33.

Terhaar, M. F., Taylor, L. A., & Sylvia, M. L. (2016). The doctor of nursing practice: From start-up to impact. *Nursing Education Perspectives, 37*(1), 3–9.

Thabane, L., Thomas, T., Ye, C., & Paul, J. (2009). Posing the research question: Not so simple. *Canadian Journal of Anesthesia, 56*(1), 71–79. doi:10.1007/s12630-008-9007-4

Thorpe, T. (2014, July 17). The top 5 reasons small businesses fail. *Inc.* Retrieved from http://www.inc.com/travis-thorpe/the-top-5-reasons-small-businesses-fail.html

Tobak, S. (2013, February 19). How to sell anything to anybody. *Inc.* Retrieved from http://www.inc.com/steve-tobak/how-to-sell-anything-to-anybody.html

Tsai, H. M., Liou, S. R., Hsiao, Y. C., & Cheng, C. Y. (2013). The relationship of individual characteristics, perceived worksite support and perceived creativity to clinical nurses' innovative outcome. *Journal of Clinical Nursing, 22*(17/18), 2648–2657.

U.S. Small Business Association. (n.d.). *Starting a business.* Retrieved from https://www.sba.gov/starting-business

United States Department of Commerce, Bureau of Economic Analysis. (2016). *National income and product accounts*. Retrieved from http://www.bea.gov/newsreleases/national/gdp/gdpnewsrelease.htm

Waddill-Goad, S. (2013). *The development of the Waddill-Goad Leadership Fatigue Questionnaire* (Doctoral dissertation). American Sentinel University, Aurora, CO.

Waddill-Goad, S. (2015, March 30 and 31). Advanced financial management: Northwest Organization of Nurse Executives (NWONE) emerging nurse leader series workshop handout.

Wagner, E. T. (2013, September 12). Five reasons 8 out of 10 businesses fail. *Forbes*. Retrieved from http://www.forbes.com/sites/ericwagner/2013/09/12/five-reasons-8-out-of-10-businesses-fail/#65864eed5e3c

Wang, J. (2016, June 1). Seven tips on entrepreneurship from America's richest self-made woman. *Forbes*. Retrieved from http://www.forbes.com/sites/jenniferwang/2016/06/01/seven-tips-on-entrepreneurship-from-americas-richest-self-made-woman/#752f2a012c74

Watson, M. (2015). Basic principles to consider when opening a nurse practitioner-owned practice in Texas. *Journal of the American Association of Nurse Practitioners, 21*(12), 683–689. doi:10.1002/2327-6924.12274

Weiss, A. (2016). *Million dollar consulting: The professional's guide to growing a practice*. New York, NY: McGraw-Hill Education.

Williams, J. (n.d.). The basics of branding. *Entrepreneur*. Retrieved from https://www.entrepreneur.com/article/77408

Wong, C. A. (2015, April). Connecting nursing leadership and patient outcomes: State of the science. *Journal of Nursing Management, 23*(3), 275–278.

The World Bank Group. (2014). *Health expenditure totals, percentage of GDP*. Retrieved from http://data.worldbank.org/indicator/SH.XPD.TOTL.ZS?locations=US

The World Bank Group. (2016). *Health expenditure totals, percentages of GDP*. Retrieved from http://data.worldbank.org/indicator/NY.GDP.PCAP.CD

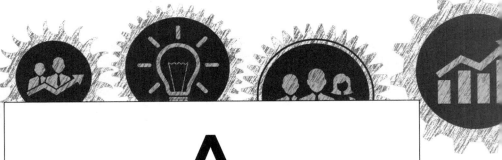

A

BASIC FINANCIAL DEFINITIONS

One of the most important things in business is to gain an understanding of finance-related concepts and terminology. It is a language unto its own. This appendix describes a number of basic concepts and their associated use in the healthcare financial arena (Waddill-Goad, 2015), in alphabetical order.

Accrual: A method of accounting that recognizes a financial or an economic event regardless of when the expense occurs.

Affordable Care Act (ACA) of 2010: A comprehensive effort to reform the current U.S. healthcare system in an attempt to improve access, reduce cost, and enhance quality. Also known as Obamacare. For an excellent summary of this legislation, visit the Kaiser Family Foundation's website: http://kff.org/health-reform/fact-sheet/summary-of-the-affordable-care-act/.

Amortization: A debt schedule paid over time.

Accounts payable: Money owed to vendors or suppliers (typically from a company) for which immediate payment is not required. Shown as unpaid invoices.

Accounts receivable: Money due from customers who have been billed for a product or service.

Asset: Any resource of value owned by a company.

Balance sheet: A financial document that provides a snapshot of a company's owned assets.

Balanced scorecard: A term used with key performance indicators (KPIs). Usually, a balanced scorecard consists of a selection of measurable items in various categories that are key to running a business.

Capacity: The people, equipment, and/or space required to produce a product or service.

Capacity utilization: An analysis and calculation (generally a percentage) of available capacity and what was actually used in the production of products and/or services.

Capital: Hard assets acquired as a long-term investment to run a business. These are noted and accounted for on a balance sheet.

Cash: Typically, a checking account balance as shown on a bank statement, currency on hand, or checks received from customers not yet deposited.

Cash flow: The movement of money in, through, and out of a company.

Consumables: Inventory consumed for the production of a service or product.

Contribution margin: A percentage that shows sales minus the cost of goods sold, divided by sales. For example, 60 – 24 = 36 / 60 = 60%. In this case, for every dollar spent, the company earns $.60.

Cost: A metric comprised of fixed, variable, flexed, direct (tied to a cost object), and indirect types of cost categories.

Cost of goods sold: The amount of money a company spends to produce a product or service.

Demand: The consumer or market need for a product or service.

Demand forecasting: The use of currently available and retrospective financial data to predict (and potentially improve) prospective or future business performance.

Depreciation: A long-term expense used to replace assets over time, equal to the expected service life of equipment. The asset value typically decreases each year.

EBITDA: Short for *earnings before interest, taxes, depreciation, and amortization.*

Equipment: Goods required to conduct business and/or the associated cost to purchase for company use.

Equity: Owned or retained earnings (usually cash) from business operations.

Expense: A cost associated with running a business.

Facility: A hard asset, such as a building, acquired or constructed by a company for its business use.

Fixed cost: Items such as labor costs/salary, overhead, and depreciation.

The Hospital Consumer Assessment of Healthcare Providers and Systems (HCAHPS): A customer-satisfaction survey used to measure patient perception of care both overall and relative to communication, responsiveness, pain management, cleanliness, and discharge, affecting certain healthcare reimbursement. Information about the survey can be found here: http://hcahpsonline.org/home.aspx.

Hospital Compare: A website that collates numerous sources for cost, clinical processes of care, patient experience, and quality data for hospitals. Comparisons are based on benchmarking (to self, achievement levels of improvement, and comparison to others). To access this site, visit https://www.medicare.gov/hospitalcompare/search.html.

Income statement: A document that shows a company's revenue, expenses, and overall profit and loss for a defined period of time.

Intangible assets: A monetary value placed on work processes, intellectual knowledge, intellectual property, etc.

Interest: The cost paid to borrow money from another entity such as a bank or other financial institution.

Inventory/stock: Items kept on hand that a company sells or uses to produce a product or service.

Invoice: A method used to charge for products or services—in other words, a bill.

Key performance indicator (KPI): A company- or industry-defined metric used to determine outcomes relative to success.

Land: A long-term cost (debt) to acquire and prepare land for use by a company in the production of products and services.

Lean: A performance-improvement methodology that uses a systematic method for eliminating waste and reducing defects.

Liability: Anything owed by a company to others, such as for purchases, money borrowed for facilities and/or land, etc.

Long-term liability: The same as a liability, but one that spans a longer period. Examples include bonds, real estate, etc.

Net profit/loss: The business's "bottom line" after all associated short-term (taxes) and long-term (interest) costs and/or expenses have been applied and accounted for in a set time period (usually monthly, quarterly, or annually).

Operating expense: A cost related to keeping a business going from day to day. These expenses are noted on the income statement.

Overhead: Non-revenue-generating cost.

Plant: Buildings and machinery used to make a product or service.

Profit: Sales or revenue minus all types of cost.

Profit and loss (P&L) statement: A document that shows the flow of value in a company, including sales and types of costs and expenses during a defined period of time.

Revenue: Payment for all services rendered (gross and net).

Return on *x*: Variable calculations to assess performance. These include return on investment, return on assets, return on capital, etc.).

Return on investment (ROI): A calculation to assess a company's cost versus the benefits it gains. Examples include ROIs for a particular type of project or equipment.

Real property: The value placed on real estate that a company owns.

Rent expense: Expenses incurred from rentals of land and/or buildings for a company's use.

Salary expenses: Expenses incurred by both hourly and salaried workers. A salaried worker's time is accounted for during an accounting period. Amounts are commonly paid as equal or fixed in weekly, bi-weekly, monthly, or annual installments. Expenses incurred by hourly workers are also usually shown and accounted for during a defined period and recorded as wage expenses.

Short-term liability: Debt settled or satisfied in the current operating cycle of a business, such as a fiscal year. Also called *current liabilities*.

Stock of materials: Items used for production of a product or service.

Stock of finished goods: Inventory yet to be sold and/or delivered to customers.

Supply: Supplies used in the production of a product or service shown in two ways: those not yet used (supply inventory) and those in use or used (expense).

Supplier: A company from which other businesses buy goods for use in the development of a product or service. Also called a *vendor*.

Supply chain: The entire process of obtaining goods to produce a product or service.

Taxes: Money paid to a governmental entity in a for-profit enterprise. The majority of hospitals are considered non-profit, meaning their profits are reinvested in the enterprise and they are not subject to numerous taxes. (This stands in contrast to for-profit hospitals, which offer distributions to shareholders, typically in the form of dividends.)

Unit of service: A measurable metric to define a business's workload.

Utility expense: A cost for electricity, water, heat, trash removal, recycling, etc. used during a specified accounting period (monthly).

Value: Describes something that has a positive effect on a business.

Value-based purchasing: The linkage of payment to a value-based system aimed at improving healthcare quality versus quantity. For more information, see https://www.cms.gov.

Variable cost: An expense that includes consumables, material used, utilities, insurance, some types of labor, etc.

Working capital: The amount of money necessary to keep a company running. It includes cash, accounts receivable, and inventory minus short-term liability (accounts payable, taxes, etc.).

Work in process/progress (WIP): A value placed on materials required for the production cycle of a product or service.

Zero-based budgeting: A prospective forecast of the future year based on the last year's actual performance. (This might also include a retrospective review of previous years.)

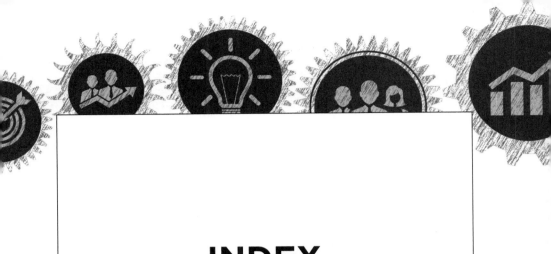

INDEX

gross domestic product (GDP), 1, 2, 5

S

T

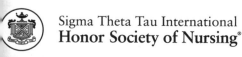
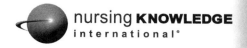

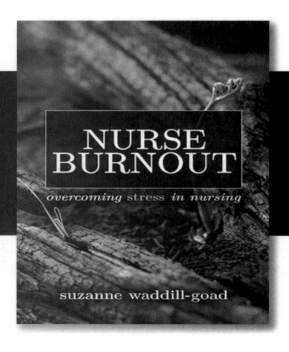
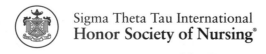
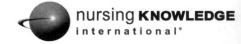

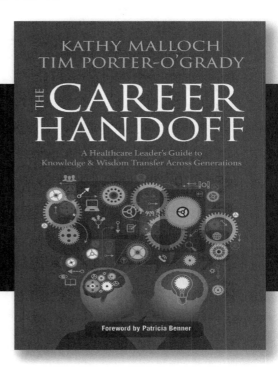
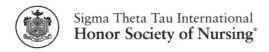
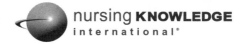

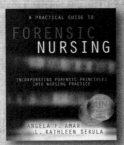
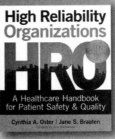
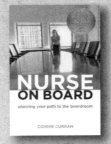
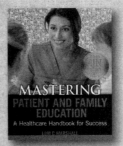